Closing India's Nutrition Gap:
The Role of Golden Mustard in Fighting
Vitamin A Deficiency

Ramanan Laxminarayan
Jeffrey Chow
Eili Klein
Paula Whitacre

RESOURCES
FOR THE FUTURE

i

Library of Congress Cataloging-in-Publication Data

Closing India's nutrition gap: the role of golden mustard in fighting vitamin A deficiency / Ramanan Laxminarayan ... [et al.].

p. ; cm.

Includes bibliographical references.

ISBN 978-1-933115-66-5 (pbk. : alk. paper) 1. Vitamin A deficiency--Treatment-- India. 2. Vitamin A deficiency--Treatment--Economic aspects--India 3. Mustard-- Therapeutic use--India. 4. Mustard oils--Therapeutic use--India.

I. Laxminarayan, Ramanan. II. Resources for the Future.

[DNLM: 1. Vitamin A Deficiency--therapy--India. 2. Dietary Supplements--economics- -India. 3. Food, Fortified--economics--India. 4. Mustard Plant--India. 5. Vitamin A Deficiency--epidemiology- -India. 6. Vitamin A Deficiency--etiology--India. WD 110 C643 2007]

RC627.V54C46 2007

613.2'860954--dc22 2007037731

Designed & Printed in India by www.shambho.in
First print: November 2007

Resources for the Future
1616 P St NW,
Washington DC 20036-1400
USA
Web: www.rff.org

About Resources for the Future (RFF)
RFF is a nonprofit and nonpartisan organization that conducts independent research—rooted primarily in economics and other social sciences—on environmental, energy, health, and natural resource issues. RFF is headquartered in Washington, DC, but its research scope comprises programs in nations around the world. Founded in 1952, RFF pioneered the application of economics as a tool to develop more effective policy for the use and conservation of natural resources. Its scholars continue to employ social science methods to analyze critical issues concerning antibiotic and anti-malarial resistance, pollution control, energy policy, land and water use, hazardous waste, climate change, and the environmental and health challenges of developing countries.

Disclaimer
The statements in this book represent the opinions of the authors; the statements do not and should not be construed to represent official policy statements or endorsements by Resources for the Future.

Contents

Abbreviations and Equivalencies

Abbreviations

DALY	disability-adjusted life year
FAO	Food and Agriculture Organization of the United Nations
GDP	gross domestic product
GM	genetically modified
HIV	human immunodeficiency virus
ICDS	Integrated Child Development Services
IOM	Institute of Medicine
IU	international unit
LHS	Latin hypercube sampling
MT	metric ton
NGO	nongovernmental organization
NNMB	National Nutrition Monitoring Bureau
PDS	Public Distribution System
RAE	retinol activity equivalent
RDA	recommended daily allowance
TPDS	Targeted Public Distribution System
USAID	U.S. Agency for International Development
USDA	U.S. Department of Agriculture
VAD	Vitamin A deficiency
WHO	World Health Organization

Equivalencies

40 rupees (Rs.) = 1 U.S. dollar ($)

1,00,000* = 100,000 = 1 lakh

100 lakhs = 1 crore

Note: Indian numeric notation will be used throughout the report.

Foreword

Micronutrient deficiencies, in the recent past, have attracted considerable attention from planners, researchers, agricultural scientists, and bureaucrats, particularly since the International Congress of Nutrition in 1992. Vitamin A deficiency is arguably the most widespread community nutrition problem in the world—in terms of the numbers of people affected. Over 220 million preschool children are estimated to be at risk of vitamin A deficiency, and at least about 3 million have xerophthalmia, eye manifestations due to vitamin A deficiency. The beneficial effect of vitamin A supplementation in reducing child mortality makes it an important public health tool to improve child survival in developing countries, particularly in Southeast Asia. National governments and international agencies like WHO, UNICEF, FAO, and USAID, among others, have been involved in serious efforts to develop suitable strategies to improve vitamin A nutriture of these populations.

Poverty, ignorance, the lack of access and availability of inexpensive micronutrient diets, and dependence on plant-based foods are major constraints for communities. And although a food-based approach and dietary diversification are undoubtedly the most logical, rational, and sustainable strategies, they require long duration to show any beneficial impact. Biannual administration of mega doses of vitamin A, if implemented properly, has been shown to be effective not only in preventing corneal xerophthalmia, but in improving child survival as well. However, the experience in India for the last 37 years indicates that there has been hardly any perceptible change in the prevalence of xerophthalmia and its consequences. This is due to poor outreach, as a result of inadequate and irregular supplies, absence of close supervision, and lack of appreciation for the importance of the programme by the health functionaries. Traditional food fortification with vitamin A has not yet been successful, despite the efforts to fortify a number of food items in different countries; its success depends upon the cooperation of the concerned industries.

Under these circumstances, this report, Closing India's Nutrition Gap: The Role of Golden Mustard in Fighting Vitamin A Deficiency by Ramanan Laxminarayan and his colleagues, discusses not only the pros and cons of bio-fortification, but also provides the readers an excellent review on the current status of various efforts to control vitamin A deficiency, particularly in India. The authors have made considerable efforts to collect and interpret observations of different aspects of vitamin A deficiency, and their critical review of literature will benefit keen students of this topic.

The authors convincingly present, with the support of scientific data and lucid analysis, the enormous potential of biofortification through adoption of appropriate methods of agricultural biotechnology. Mustard oil is consumed extensively in certain northern and eastern parts of India, and biofortification of the oil has enormous potential to improve the vitamin A status of the populations in these areas. Since these populations are socio-economically poor and have widespread vitamin A deficiency, biofortification could be an important public health tool in the future.

This publication could be considered as a compendium on public health aspects of vitamin A deficiency. The chapter on cost-effectiveness analysis—through a study of the relative efficiency of biofortified mustard, as compared to supplementation and fortification of mustard oil during processing for treating vitamin A deficiency in India—is an important highlight of the publication. The extensive analysis, based on data from 16 states where mustard is grown and consumed, includes calculations of avertable disease burden in terms of Disability Adjusted Life Years (DALYs). The presentation is not only scientific, but is an honest interpretation of the cost-effectiveness of the various approaches. For students of community nutrition and community health, this chapter is very informative and could serve even as a guide for future such studies with different strategies.

Of course, it should be recognized that such an analysis is also based on certain assumptions, whenever scientific data is not available, and to that extent, one could argue that the results could be vitiated. Another limitation, which has been pointed out, is that vitamin A deficiency is not a public health problem in some of the states included in this study. Nevertheless, the comparisons will remain valid, as such limitations are common to all the strategies compared.

The advantages of golden mustard are that in the areas where it is consumed, all the segments of the population avail themselves of the benefit, and more importantly, consumption is independent of external factors like inadequate supplies, and is not personnel-dependent like the present supplementary programmes of either vitamin A or iron folic acid. Consumption, however, is dependent on the cost of the product, and it is yet to be seen as to what proportion of the needy really has access to it. The attitudes and the policies of the government, with respect to genetically modified (GM) foods, can also influence production and consumption of golden mustard. The safety aspects of all GM foods are important, and appropriate quality assurance measures should be developed simultaneously. The safety aspects are emphasized by the Indian Health and Family Welfare Ministry under the Prevention of Food Adulteration Act, which calls for mandatory labeling. Golden mustard could open the gates for scientific advances in the field of agricultural biotechnology so as to benefit the community at large.

This report will definitely be of considerable use, not only to academics and scientists working in the area, but also to administrators and policymakers. The authors deserve congratulations for their efforts. I am sure that it will receive critical acclaim from academics and planners alike.

16-09-2007   Dr. K. Vijayaraghavan
                                         Former Senior Deputy Director, NIN
                                              Director Research, SHARE India,
                                        Mediciti Institute of Medical Sciences,
                                                         Hyderabad, India

Acknowledgments

This report was prepared by a team led by Ramanan Laxminarayan, Senior Fellow, Resources for the Future (RFF) and comprised of Jeffrey Chow, Research Associate, RFF; Eili Klein, Research Assistant, RFF; and Paula Whitacre, independent consultant. The report benefited from consultations with the following individuals:

Gerard Barry, International Rice Research Institute
Ramesh Bhat, National Institute of Nutrition
G.N.V. Brahmam, National Institute of Nutrition
Saraswathi Bulusu, Micronutrient Initiative
Vibha Dhawan, The Energy and Resources Institute
Cherian George, Monsanto Company
Rajan Kapoor, Monsanto Company
Anand Lakshman, Micronutrient Initiative
Rakesh Mittal, Indian Council for Medical Research
S.R. Rao, Department of Biotechnology, Government of India
H.B. Singh, Mustard Research and Promotion Council
Mani Subramiyam, Centre for Development Research and Training
G.S. Toteja, Indian Council for Medical Research
Kamasamudram Vijayaraghavan, National Institute of Nutrition
Satyajeet Yadav, Mustard Research and Promotion Council

These individuals provided substantive and valuable input to the report, but they were not asked to endorse its conclusions and did not see the final version before it was published. The authors bear full responsibility for the final content.

The report was edited by Sally Atwater under the direction of Felicia Day and Adrienne Foerster. Sarah Darley managed overall report production. Janet Carpenter, U.S. Agency for International Development, provided useful guidance throughout the course of the project. Cover photograph of mustard flower by Utsav Arora. Cover photograph of Rajasthani mother and child by David Zimmerly.

The report was produced under a grant from the International Center for Tropical Agriculture (CIAT), Colombia.

Executive Summary

Humans need vitamin A for such essential processes as growth, vision, and resistance to infectious disease. Vitamin A deficiency (VAD) arises from prolonged inadequate intake combined with periods of higher physiological demand, such as during childhood growth spurts, pregnancy, and lactation, or through increased utilization during infection (Sommer and West 1996). Thus, young children and pregnant and lactating women are at greatest risk and are the most common victims. It occurs primarily among people with limited food choices, particularly those in the lower socioeconomic strata of poor countries with diets predominated by less nutritious staple foods (Sommer and West 1996).

VAD is a significant cause of blindness and death. It also has economic implications. Improving a person's nutritional status can result in an increase in lifetime earnings of at least 10 percent. Taken collectively, a population's nutritional status can make a difference of 2 to 3 percent in a country's gross domestic product. Conversely, about 5 percent of the gross national product of South Asia is lost each year because of deficiencies in the intakes of vitamin A, iron, and iodine (World Bank 2005).

Vitamin A in food is available as retinol in animal foods, such as meat, dairy products, and breast milk, or as carotenoids, present in many fruits and vegetables. It is much more efficiently absorbed in the body through animal rather than plant foods (IOM 2000). Although absorption varies, depending on a person's existing stores, the method of food preparation, and other factors, people who rely on vegetables and fruits for their vitamin A intake may not get sufficient amounts through normal food consumption.

Women and especially children under age 5 have been the focus of worldwide efforts to improve vitamin A status, including periodic high-dosage supplementation, vitamin A fortification of commonly eaten foods, and other food-based approaches, such as nutrition education and home gardening programs. These efforts, challenging to implement in any country, have had a very limited reach in India. Supplementation programs face unique challenges in the Indian context, related to poor coverage by immunization programs and the lack of recognition of the public health importance of VAD by many in the scientific community and government. Fortification has had limited success because of the large number of small manufacturers of food and a regulatory system not strong enough to enforce fortification rules. And other food-based approaches have not made significant inroads in a country with very diverse agricultural conditions and dietary patterns.

Because of those limitations, new approaches may be needed to reduce VAD in India. In recent years, the Monsanto Company and The Energy and Resource Institute have developed innovative methods involving genetic recombinant technology to biofortify mustard, the source of a commonly used cooking and pickling oil in many states in northern India, where VAD prevalence is high, to increase its vitamin A content. This technology, like that used to develop biofortified or "golden" rice[1], can fortify mustard to a far greater extent than is possible through traditional methods of fortification.

This publication begins to answer some of the questions that arise about the feasibility of further development of this technology. We focus on whether mustard production and consumption patterns indicate the appropriateness of mustard oil as a vehicle to increase vitamin A intake in target groups of lower-income children and pregnant and lactating women. Further, we present results of our analysis of the cost-effectiveness of biofortified mustard compared with high-dosage supplementation and traditional fortification of foods.

The Landscape of Vitamin A Deficiency

Recognition of the ocular consequences of a VAD evolved over many centuries. It was not until the 1980s, however, that broader impacts on morbidity and mortality were confirmed, when a community trial in the 1980s demonstrated a 34 percent reduction in mortality for preschool children (aged 12–71 months) and a 26 percent reduction for all children who were given vitamin A supplements, compared with a control group (Sommer, Djunaedi et al. 1986). Subsequent studies reported less dramatic findings, yet a broad scientific consensus has emerged that vitamin A likely confers protective effects on health, resulting in lower levels of mortality, most likely through the reduction in the duration of disease (Grotto, Mimouni et al. 2003).

VAD is ideally measured by the level of serum retinol in the blood and liver. However, such tests are expensive and difficult to administer in areas with limited health services. As a result, the World Health Organization (WHO) has established other indicators to determine the extent and severity of VAD in a country or region. They include functional indicators (e.g., night blindness and foamy white spots on the cornea known as Bitot's spots), as well as "non-specific but supportive ecologic and demographic" indicators, such as mortality rates, dietary patterns, disease prevalence, and income levels (WHO 1996).

WHO considers VAD a public health challenge in more than 100 countries worldwide (Rice, West Jr. et al. 2004), mostly in Africa and South Asia, affecting more than 25 crore (250 million) preschool children. Between 2,50,000 and 5,00,000 children lose their sight each year (WHO 2006). Approximately 72 lakh (7.2 million) pregnant women in developing countries are vitamin A deficient, as estimated from serum retinol levels, and more than 60 lakh (6 million) develop night blindness each year (Rice, West Jr. et al. 2004).

Within South Asia, 40 percent of children from birth to age 4 suffer from VAD, the highest percentage of any region in the world (Rice, West Jr. et al. 2004). This region-wide figure, however, masks disparities between countries, with India having by far the highest rate of subclinical VAD and among the highest rate of clinical VAD in the region. Each year, VAD is associated with the deaths of 3,33,000 children in India (Gragnolati, Shekar et al. 2005). Although improvements in vitamin A status have been noted during the past two decades, as late as the 1990s only 11 percent of the population in a survey conducted by India's National Nutrition Monitoring Bureau (NNMB) had adequate intake of vitamin A (NNMB 2000). Most of those surveyed consumed less than 30 percent of the recommended levels, and 57 percent of children and 5 percent of pregnant women were vitamin A deficient.

The severity of VAD varies across and within states. The positive news is that clinical VAD has generally declined in India over the past 30 years, as indicated by a decreased prevalence of Bitot's spots among young children in rural areas. However, it remains a persistent problem (Toteja and Singh 2004), and more recent data suggest a possible resurgence (Mason, Bailes et al. 2005). In most age groups, it affects a slightly higher percentage of females. In both rural and urban areas, households with the lowest income per capita typically consume the least amounts of vitamin A, as well as other essential micronutrients, such as iron, iodine, and zinc.

Addressing Vitamin A Deficiencies

Chapter 2 reviews India's experiences with the three most commonly used interventions to address VAD: high-dosage supplementation, food fortification, and other food-based approaches, such as dietary diversification.

Supplementation. In 1970, India launched one of the world's first supplementation programs as a method to prevent blindness. However, coverage of children in India remains low. In 2000, it was estimated that only about 31 percent of children between 9 and 12 months old received vitamin A supplementation (Vijayaraghavan 2006). A much-publicized case in Assam in 2001, in which more than 14 children died after participating in a supplementation program, may have depressed coverage further since then. In addition, supplementation is not universally supported by India's medical establishment. For example, the 2000 National Consultation on the Benefits and Safety of Vitamin A Administration concluded that "available data are not robust enough to persuade us to recommend a policy of vitamin A supplementation for the purpose of mortality reduction in children" (National Consultation 2001), although the panel did not recommend ending the program.

Fortification. Fortification, a process in which vitamin A (and/or other nutrients) is added to commonly consumed foods, offers an opportunity to improve micronutrient status without changing food habits. It also expands coverage to people who would not normally receive supplementation but who are at risk, such as women and older children.

To be effective, the product to be fortified must be centrally processed, and fortification must be regulated, monitored, and marketed. One of the most successful examples to date is fortification of sugar in Central America, but few other centrally processed foods have such widespread reach. Less than 1 percent of food in India is fortified, despite many innovative attempts and pilot projects. India has many mechanisms that could be used to distribute fortified foods, such as the Public Distribution System and the Targeted Public Distribution System. However, the dispersed nature of food production, combined with the large variety in food preferences, means that vitamin A-fortified foods are not routinely consumed in much of India.

Food-based approaches. As a third strategy to increase vitamin A intake, people can be educated and encouraged to consume more vitamin A-rich foods. Some promising projects include a home gardening project in Andhra Pradesh, nutrition education through the National Institute of Nutrition, and efforts to increase consumption of red palm oil, which is particularly high in beta-carotene. At this point, however, these approaches have not measurably improved the vitamin A status of the targeted vulnerable populations in India, particularly lower-income children and women.

Mustard and Its Potential to Reduce Vitamin A Deficiency in India

As reported in Chapter 3, mustard and rapeseed crops (the two are combined in most agricultural statistics) account for about 22 percent of India's oilseed production. About 90 percent of mustard is processed into oil for cooking and pickling.

About 90 percent of the 4 to 5 crore (40 to 50 million) farmers who grow mustard in India do so on a very small scale. Mustard production is centered in the north, with Rajasthan as the largest producing state. Farmers generally purchase new seed each year, typically at melas (farm fairs), which are also a source of general agricultural information.

In ascending order of efficiency and yield, oil from mustard seed is processed at home with a mortar and pestle, in village-based mills (ghanis), at small-scale expeller facilities, and by large manufacturers. Large companies, primarily in Rajasthan, Uttar Pradesh, Haryana, and Punjab, account for around 75 percent of total production, although in terms of numbers of facilities, ghanis are the most numerous (1,50,000).

Mustard oil has a shelf life of up to one year but is seldom kept that long before consumption. However, proper storage is an important issue. Because light breaks down vitamin A, mustard oil, if made from biofortified seed, would need to be transported and stored in sealed, dark containers.

Mustard oil is a fairly integral part of many northern Indian households, regardless of income (Dohlman, Persaud et al. 2003), in both rural and urban areas. It is purchased in small quantities from bulk suppliers or packaged as branded oil. Assuming that all oil were biofortified and cooking did not reduce the amount of beta-carotene in the oil (both overly optimistic assumptions), a child would need 1 to 4 grams of oil per day (about a teaspoon) to meet the full recommended daily allowance, with no other sources of vitamin A. However, most children consume at least some amount of vitamin A from other sources, which suggests that even if the beta-carotene content in the oil were lower, small dosages could still increase intake to recommended daily levels.

Development of a transgenic canola plant, a close botanical relative of mustard, has resulted in a 50-fold increase in carotenoids (Shewmaker, Sheehy et al. 1999). Research to develop transgenic lines of Indian mustard has shown promise, although challenges remain. To date, only about 1 per 100 plants has been successfully transformed, and both genetically modified (GM) mustard and canola seeds have slightly lower yields than their conventional counterparts. In addition, India's political and legal environment for genetically modified plants must be taken into account.

Cost-Effectiveness Analysis for Treating Vitamin A Deficiency in India

Chapter 4 presents an analysis of the relative efficiency of biofortified mustard, compared with supplementation and fortification of mustard oil during processing. We compared the three strategies by calculating avertable disease burden in terms of disability-adjusted life years (DALYs)[2] and by comparing cost-effectiveness ratios in terms of unit cost per DALY averted over a 20-year time frame.

The analysis looked at 16 states that grow and/or consume mustard, in eight of which (Assam, Bihar, Jharkland, Madhya Pradesh, Rajasthan, Uttar Pradesh, and Tripura), as shown through prevalence of Bitot's spots, vitamin A consumption is insufficient. Each intervention was evaluated according to the ratio of its total cost to total effectiveness. A greater cost-effectiveness ratio indicates a higher cost per unit of health gained. (In other words, a high ratio indicates low efficiency or less cost-effectiveness, and a low ratio indicates the opposite.) An internal rate of return was also calculated for each intervention, although we stress that the internal rates of return are for comparative purposes only and do not predict rates of return on investments.

The analysis shows that the most cost-effective intervention remains supplementation, at approximately Rs. 930–1,500 per DALY averted, followed by biofortification (Rs. 3,660–8,410 per DALY averted) and traditional fortification (Rs. 6,880–10,060 per DALY averted). The internal rate of return for supplementation far exceeds that of either fortification or biofortification: 82–104 percent for supplementation, compared with an internal rate of return of 11–22 percent for fortification and 16–43 percent for biofortification.

Despite less favorable cost-effectiveness ratios and internal rate of return numbers, however, fortification and biofortification reach a wider number of women and children than supplementation. Biofortification has the potential to avert the greatest burden of deaths due to VAD. We estimate that biofortification could avert 1.5–3.4 crore DALYs and 2.8–6.5 lakh deaths, and traditional fortification could avert 1.3–1.9 crore DALYs and 1.6–3.6 lakh deaths over a 20-year period. In contrast, while vitamin A supplementation targeted at preschool children in mustard-consuming states could avert 1.7–2.8 crore DALYs and approximately 2.6–6 lakh childhood deaths, without expansion of health subcenter coverage, these numbers fall to only 44–71 lakh DALYs and 68,000–1,58,000 deaths averted over the 20-year period.

The disadvantage of traditional fortification of oil is the need for effective monitoring and enforcement, which is feasible only in the larger processing facilities. In contrast, biofortification of mustard seed is an attractive alternative in most of the states analyzed. Farmers purchase new seed yearly, and fortification of the seed gets around the problem of highly decentralized oil-processing facilities. A program to support, monitor, and enforce biofortification could efficiently yield substantial improvements in health in states where mustard oil is consumed, especially in states where VAD constitutes a public health problem and a lot of oil is produced.

Despite its potential, biofortified mustard oil comes with a unique set of hurdles. Introduction of GM food products may require additional costs for education and awareness campaigns, and the attitude of Indians toward GM food and agriculture is mixed. Although these considerations are outside the scope of this study, they must be taken into account in decisions to allocate resources toward biofortification of mustard seed.

Conclusions and Recommendations

The final section of this report presents the conclusions and recommendations reached through our analysis.

1. The public health significance of vitamin A deficiency is underrecognized in India. Without greater emphasis on VAD by India's premier medical institutions, it will be difficult to gather momentum around any strategy to address the problem.

2. Supplementation, fortification, and food-based approaches have been relatively unsuccessful for operational, social, and political reasons. The current supplementation program reaches only about one-third of the children who need it. Fortification is hampered by lack of enforcement, resistance from producers, and the dispersed nature of food production and processing. Food-based approaches have not had much impact because of low levels of consumption of animal products in lower-income households.

3. Biofortification can be a cost-effective way to reach severely vitamin A-deficient households. Since biofortification does not depend on industry cooperation (unlike traditional fortification), does not require an operational infrastructure for delivery (unlike supplementation), and can provide extremely high levels of beta-carotene (unlike many food-based approaches), it can sidestep the hurdles other methods face in addressing VAD.

4. Important operational challenges of implementing biofortification will have to be addressed. Biofortification requires that farmers adopt GM mustard varieties and that consumers pay for oil that may look different. Vertically integrated approaches that combine mustard growing, oil extraction, and targeting to high-risk consumers are likely to be very resource intensive. A lower level of investment is needed for market-based approaches that only subsidize mustard seeds, but these approaches may not have much impact unless the biofortified mustard varieties are adopted widely.

5. The optimal approach to addressing VAD in India is likely a mix of strategies. Because each strategy has advantages and disadvantages, and because cultural and socioeconomic conditions vary across the country, a combination of approaches may offer the best chances of success. In mustard-consuming states at least, biofortification has the potential to substantially reduce VAD. States that do not consume mustard oil, however, must continue to rely on supplementation to improve their vitamin A status or else develop an appropriate alternative fortification vehicle. Efforts to further test the technological and economic feasibility of biofortified mustard, possibly leading to commercial production, must take these broader considerations into account.

Notes

[1] Beta-carotene has a reddish-yellowish tinge that, when super-concentrated in GM rice or mustard, turns it a golden color.

[2] DALYs are a measure of healthy life years: the sum of the present value of years of future lifetime lost through premature mortality, and the present value of years of future lifetime adjusted for the average severity of the mental or physical disability caused by a disease or injury (Rushby and Hanson 2001).

Introduction

Vitamin A is a class of fat-soluble molecules with the structure of retinoids and biologic activity comparable to retinol (West and Darnton-Hill 2001). It occurs naturally in animal foods, such as eggs and dairy products, and as carotenoids (provitamin A, beta-carotene in particular) in plant sources, such as yellow fruits and dark green leafy vegetables. Vitamin A is necessary for many physiological processes, including morphogenesis, growth, vision, reproduction, cellular differentiation, and resistance to infectious disease. An essential nutrient, vitamin A cannot be synthesized in humans—it must come from dietary intake of active or precursor forms.

Vitamin A deficiency (VAD) arises from prolonged inadequate intake combined with periods of higher physiological demand, such as during childhood growth spurts, pregnancy, and lactation, or through increased utilization during infection (Sommer and West 1996). Thus, young children and pregnant and lactating women are at greatest risk and are the most common VAD victims. VAD occurs primarily among people with limited food choices, particularly those in the lower socioeconomic strata of poor countries with diets predominated by less nutritious staple foods (Sommer and West 1996). Women and especially children under age 5 have been the focus of worldwide efforts to improve vitamin A status. These efforts have included periodic high-dosage supplementation, vitamin A fortification of commonly eaten foods, and other food-based approaches, such as nutrition education and home gardening programs.

VAD is a significant cause of blindness and death in India. Although improvements in vitamin A status have been noted during the past 2 decades (NNMB 2000), as late as the 1990s only 11 percent of the population in a survey conducted by India's National Nutrition Monitoring Bureau (NNMB) had adequate intake of vitamin A. Most of those surveyed consumed less than 30 percent of the recommended levels, and 57 percent of children and 5 percent of pregnant women were vitamin A deficient. The South Asia region has among the highest rates in the world, and India leads the region, in both the percentage and the total number of children who have VAD, as well as in the number of maternal xerophthalmia cases (West Jr. 2002). Each year, VAD is associated with the death of 3,33,000 children in India (Gragnolati, Shekar et al. 2005).

The challenges of delivering vitamin A to those who need it are especially significant in India. VAD populations tend to be geographically dispersed and difficult to identify and reach. Poverty is often cited as an important reason why VAD persists in India. It is not a full explanation, however, since other countries in the region with similar socioeconomic profiles have made significant strides in reducing VAD prevalence, largely through supplementation and fortification programs. Supplementation programs face unique challenges in the Indian context, specifically related to poor coverage by immunization programs and the lack of recognition of the public health importance of VAD by both the scientific community and the government. Fortification methods have had limited success because there are many small manufacturers of food and the regulatory system is not strong enough to enforce fortification rules. And other food-based approaches have not made significant inroads in a country with very diverse agricultural conditions and dietary patterns.

Because of those limitations, new approaches may be needed to reduce VAD in India. In recent years, innovative methods involving genetic recombinant technology have been developed to biofortify mustard, the source of a commonly used cooking and pickling oil in many Indian states where VAD prevalence is high, to increase its vitamin A content. This technology can fortify mustard to a greater extent than is possible through traditional methods of fortification.

In this study, we evaluate different strategies for reducing VAD in India, including supplementation programs, fortification, and biofortification, with an emphasis on evaluating the potential for biofortification. Answers to the following questions will determine whether mustard biofortification has a useful role to play in India's public health campaign. How does biofortification compare with traditional methods of fortification and supplementation? Are the people who consume mustard oil the same as those who have the highest levels of VAD? Would growing and distributing biofortified mustard result in increased vitamin A intake by those who need it most? What kinds of economic incentives would be required to produce and encourage the consumption of biofortified mustard, and would the costs be worth the potential health benefits? What strategies would ensure that biofortified mustard oil reaches the most deficient populations? How could current mustard growing and processing systems accommodate the introduction of biofortified seed?

In addressing these questions, we have made several assumptions. First, we assume that research into biofortified mustard conducted by the

Monsanto Corporation and The Energy and Resource Institute in India (TERI) can ultimately produce a safe mustard variety appropriate to Indian growing conditions. We further assume that government policies would allow for the distribution of these seeds to farmers who currently grow conventional mustard or who may be interested in growing a new crop. Finally, although public debate about the safety of genetically modified (GM) foods is ongoing in many countries, analyzing this debate and its impact in India is not within the scope of this report.

We have organized this study as follows. After an overview of the prevalence and consequences of VAD in Chapter 1, we summarize how supplementation, fortification, and food-based approaches are used in India and in other countries in Chapter 2. Chapter 3 turns to an examination of current mustard production and consumption in India, including whether biofortified mustard can be an appropriate vehicle to increase vitamin A intake in target groups. The main part of the analysis comes in Chapter 4, where we present a cost-effectiveness analysis that compares biofortified mustard with high-dosage supplementation and traditional fortification. In the final section, we summarize our conclusions and recommendations.

Our main finding is that under some conditions, a biofortification strategy can play an important role as part of a broader approach to reducing VAD prevalence in India. Biofortification strategies can be cost-effective, feasible, and implemented under conditions where supplementation and fortification are currently disadvantaged. There are some significant barriers, however. First, there is insufficient recognition of the importance of VAD as a public health problem in India. Many in the medical and scientific community remain unconvinced of the mortality effects of VAD. Without a move toward scientific consensus on the urgent need to address VAD, all strategies to address VAD are doomed to failure. Second, in addition to technological and market-related issues associated with GM agricultural products, concerns about the safety of GM mustard (also known as biofortified or "golden" mustard, terms used interchangeably), or indeed any GM food, to human health and the environment remains a continuing barrier to wider adoption. These issues are outside the scope of this report.

Additional technological risks are associated with growing a mustard variety that has been genetically modified to express a higher level of beta-carotene. One theoretical possibility is that in certain conditions, the modified variety is inherently inferior to the traditional varieties, but presumably higher susceptibility to frost or other weaknesses would be discovered and overcome during field trials. Similarly, there could be a yield loss, currently of unknown magnitude, associated with biofortified crops, which again would likely be revealed in field trials. Moreover, lower-probability events, such as pest outbreaks, could put the GM mustard at greater risk than conventional varieties. Although we do not formally analyze technological risks, we discuss some potential risks in this report. Finally, there are issues related to consumer acceptability of a new technology. Although GM foods do not face skepticism and negative response from consumers in India to the same extent that they do in Europe and other parts of the world, the acceptability of biofortified mustard oil remains to be seen.

Those concerns notwithstanding, biofortification technologies have enormous potential for delivering micronutrients to regions and populations where traditional methods of supplementation and fortification have been unsuccessful. Although the largest numbers of people affected with VAD live in India, VAD is a public health problem in more than 100 countries worldwide (Rice, West Jr. et al. 2004), mostly in Africa and Asia. Although most successes in agricultural biotechnology worldwide to date have been in pest protection and other yield-enhancing benefits to commercial crops, its great promise lies in addressing nutritional deficiencies. This study, although specific to a single crop in India, offers some insight into the advantages and challenges faced by agricultural biotechnology-based strategies to address nutritional deficiencies in other parts of the world.

CHAPTER 1

The Landscape of Vitamin A Deficiency in India

Since ancient times, healers and other observers have made a connection between certain foods and unique ocular problems, such as night blindness and corneal destruction, termed xerophthalmia[1], making vitamin A deficiency one of the world's oldest recorded medical problems. Ocular issues, though, are just the end stage of the deficiency. VAD is also associated with retarded growth, increased susceptibility to diseases, and increased mortality. However, VAD was not identified as a major public health problem in the developing world until the 1980s, when researchers demonstrated the clear link between a lack of vitamin A and increased morbidity and mortality.

Currently, VAD is considered a public health challenge in more than 100 countries worldwide (Rice, West Jr. et al. 2004), mostly in Africa and South Asia. The World Health Organization (WHO) estimates that more than 25 crore (250 million) preschool children and a substantial number of pregnant women are vitamin A deficient, and as a result, 2,50,000 to 5,00,000 lose their sight each year (WHO 2006). Despite significant progress over the past several years, the largest number of these VAD children and expectant mothers live in India (West Jr. 2002).

In this chapter, we focus on the scope of the problem, including where and among whom in India VAD poses the greatest threat. We also briefly discuss the consequences of VAD when people do not consume the recommended daily amounts of this essential nutrient.

History

Recognition of the ocular consequences of a VAD evolved over many centuries. In ancient Egypt and Greece, it was separately observed that a piece of animal liver, either placed on top of the eyes or consumed, could treat destructive eye problems (Wolf 1996). Physicians in the 17th and 18th centuries noted the connection between severe protein malnutrition and corneal destruction resulting in permanent blindness. By the late 1800s, doctors had recognized and routinely recommended that meat, milk, and cod liver oil could cure night blindness and Bitot's spots (Sommer and West 1996), the foamy white spots on the cornea first described by the French physician Pierre Bitot. In the early 20th century, robust scientific investigation of the role of nutrition and health led to E.V. McCollum's identification of the essential role that vitamin A plays in growth and immune systems by studying the absence or presence of what was then called fat-soluble factor A in rats (Underwood 2004). Later identified as retinol, this fat-soluble nutrient is stored in the liver, where a person can accumulate significant stores of vitamin A.

By the 1920s, the cause and the cure for VAD were well established, and it soon ceased to be a problem for most countries of the developed world (Sommer and West 1996). Elsewhere, however, despite significant evidence that xerophthalmia was a serious problem, especially in South and East Asia, public health agencies did little to intervene. Outside institutions and governments, though well intentioned, were unable to marshal significant support to increase vitamin A consumption (Reddy 2002a). The stepped-up effort of the past few decades stems in large part from a community trial in the 1980s that demonstrated a 34 percent reduction in mortality for preschool children aged 12–71 months and a 26 percent reduction for all children who were given vitamin A supplements, compared with a control group (Sommer, Djunaedi et al. 1986). Following the publication of this study and promotion by the United Nations Subcommittee on Nutrition, vitamin A supplementation began to be taken seriously by public health agencies, and follow-up studies were conducted around the developing world.

A meta-analysis of studies suggested that supplementation with high doses of vitamin A could reduce mortality rates approximately 23 percent (95 percent confidence interval [CI]: 12 to 32 percent) (Beaton, Martorell et al. 1994). Yet other studies have found little or no effect of vitamin A on mortality (Cohen, Rahman et al. 1987; Vijayaraghavan, Radhaiah et al. 1990; Herrera, Nestel et al. 1992). In a more recent study conducted in northern India, reductions in mortality were much lower–about 4 percent (95 percent CI:–3 to 11 percent), which the study authors suggest implies that reductions in mortality from vitamin A supplementation may be only 10 to 15 percent–though are likely still significant (Awasthi, Peto et al. 2007). All of these studies together suggest that vitamin A supplementation alone may not be enough to reduce mortality or morbidity, but must be combined with other measures to reduce poverty, improve sanitation, and increase dietary intake of multiple micronutrients. Additional studies have indicated that other micronutrients may increase the absorption potential of vitamin A (Dijkhuizen, Wieringa et al. 2004) and that smaller but more frequent doses of vitamin A may be more beneficial than one high dose (Humphrey, West Jr. et al. 1993), such that differing factors, such as diet, account for the divergent results. A 2003 study, though, recommended supplementation only in communities where VAD exists because high-dose vitamin A supplementation may actually be detrimental to those with adequate stores of the vitamin (Grotto, Mimouni et al. 2003).

Despite those conflicting studies, there remains a broad scientific consensus that adequate stores of vitamin A likely confer some protective effect on health. The observed lower levels of mortality are most likely attributable to the reduction in duration of disease (Grotto, Mimouni et al. 2003), though the reduction amount varies based on prior levels in the body as well as other factors, such as diet. Despite the uncertainty surrounding the resultant efficacy of high-dose vitamin A supplementation on mortality, there is consensus that supplementation reduces the likelihood of xerophthalmia when administered to those who are not receiving enough vitamin A through their diet.

The Extent of Vitamin A Deficiency

Measurements of retinol in the blood (serum retinol level) can identify VAD. Ideally, however, because individuals store vitamin A in the liver, measurement of an individual's total body stores of retinol (in both the blood and the liver) is the most accurate subclinical indicator of VAD. In developing countries, neither measurement is widely used because of the cost and lack of health services. Instead, VAD in individuals is typically diagnosed through examination for clinical symptoms, generally night blindness and Bitot's spots. This method, however, misses those who suffer from subclinical VAD and may have increased susceptibility to disease and childhood mortality.

The WHO has established several indicators to determine the extent and severity of VAD in a country or region, in addition to the functional (e.g., Bitot's spots and night blindness) and biochemical (e.g., serum retinol levels) indicators mentioned above. They include "non-specific but supportive ecologic and demographic" indicators, such as mortality rates, dietary patterns, disease prevalence, and income levels (WHO 1996).

WHO recommends that VAD be considered a public health problem in a country or region where more than 1 percent of children under age 6 suffer from night blindness or 0.5 percent from Bitot's spots. However, identifying VAD, especially subclinical VAD, is not always easy. Although it is fairly easy to identify children suffering from night blindness, Bitot's spots, or other sequelae, those with low serum retinol levels but no outward clinical symptoms may also be at risk. In addition, the regions where VAD is a problem tend to be poorer and more remote areas or urban slums; thus, data even on clinical levels of VAD are difficult to obtain. For these reasons, where these data are not available, WHO suggests that an under-5 mortality rate of more than 70 per 1,000 indicates that VAD is of concern. The International Vitamin A Consultative Group (a group of vitamin A researchers now part of a broader Micronutrient Forum, http://ivacg.ilsi. org/) suggests a lower rate, stating that an under-5 morality rate of more than 50 per 1,000 indicates a VAD problem, and a rate between 20 and 50 indicates that the area warrants further assessment (IVACG 2002). The International Vitamin A Consultative Group also considers VAD a public health priority where more than 5 percent of women had night blindness during their most recent pregnancy.

Worldwide

The number of children and women affected by VAD can be measured in multiples of crores, although the range of estimates varies considerably, in part because of the complexity of the measurement task and the paucity of data in many countries. In 1995, the WHO and the United Nations Children's Fund (UNICEF) estimated that 25.4 crore (254 million) children had VAD disorders and 28 lakh (2.8 million) children had clinical VAD (WHO 1995)[2]. More recently, it was estimated that some 12.7 crore (127 million) children had VAD disorders and 44 lakh (4.4 million) children had clinical VAD (West Jr. 2002).

Every year, an estimated 2,50,000 to 5,00,000 vitamin A-deficient children become blind, and more than half of them die within 12 months of losing their sight (WHO 2006). VAD also increases a child's risk of dying from other diseases (see Health Impacts, below): estimates suggest that VAD results in the death of 12–30 lakh (1.2–3 million) children each year (UNICEF/Micronutrient Initiative 2004).

Approximately 72 lakh (7.2 million) pregnant women in developing countries are vitamin A deficient, as estimated from serum retinol levels, and more than 60 lakh (6 million) develop night blindness each year. This represents almost 7 percent of the estimated 10.7 crore (107 million) women who annually give birth in these areas (Rice, West Jr. et al. 2004), which implies that their infants are also likely born in an already compromised state.

South Asia

Roughly 45 percent of vitamin A-deficient children and pregnant women live in South and Southeast Asia (West Jr. 2002). Within just South Asia, 40 percent of young children from birth through age 4 suffer from VAD, the highest percentage of any region in the world (Rice, West Jr. et al. 2004). This region-wide figure, however, masks wide disparities between countries, with India having by far the highest rate of subclinical VAD in the region (Figure 1-1). India also has one of the highest rates of clinical VAD in the region (Figure 1-2); moreover, it jumped by 0.5 percent in five years, from 1.2 percent in 1995 to 1.7 percent in 2000 (not pictured).

Figure 1-1. Prevalence of Subclinical VAD in Children Aged 0–72 Months in South and Southeast Asia, 2000

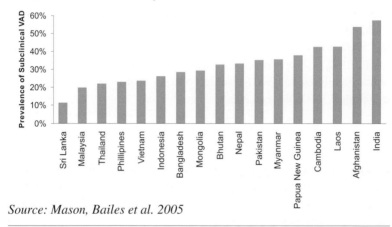

Source: Mason, Bailes et al. 2005

Figure 1-2. Prevalence of Clinical VAD in Children Aged 0–72 Months in South and Southeast Asia, 2000

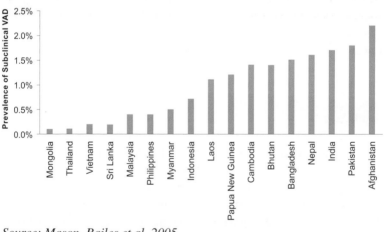

Source: Mason, Bailes et al. 2005

Why does South Asia, and India in particular, have such high prevalence rates of VAD? The underlying reasons are not entirely clear. Expected factors, such as poverty, food supply, and inequalities, do not seem to fully explain these high rates (Ramalingaswami, Jonsson et al. 1997). Poverty plays a role, but poverty rates in South Asia are lower than in sub-Saharan Africa. Fairly large food surpluses due to the Green Revolution in India and similar efforts elsewhere in South Asia suggest that the food supply is adequate. Inequalities do play a role, but they are generally no worse than in other parts of the developing world (Bhutta 2000). Some researchers have suggested that there is a more significant divide in mortality based on gender in South Asia (Ahmed, Azim et al. 2003) and India in particular (Subramanian, Nandy et al. 2006). These studies suggest that females in South Asia are routinely more likely to be underweight than males, which impairs their ability to nurture their children. The result is a high proportion of low-birth-weight babies, who are more likely to suffer from malnutrition and other significant problems during their first two years of life. These studies also point out that almost 60 percent of children are underweight before age 2 (Figure 1-3)—a formative time in childhood development—yet India's principal health program for children, the Integrated Child Development Services (ICDS), reaches only 50 to 60 percent of children and usually not until they are about 2 years old (see Box 2-3 in Chapter 2).

Figure 1-3. Prevalence of Indian Children under 3 who are Underweight

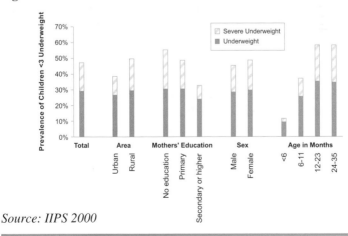

Source: IIPS 2000

India

National Overview

Even with incomplete data, it is clear that India has the most vitamin A-deficient children in the region and among the highest numbers in the world, as well as the largest number of maternal xerophthalmia cases (West Jr. 2002). Population size, of course, contributes to these high numbers: the number of people who live on less than Rs. 40 (US$1) per day—44 crore (440 million) people, or 44 percent of the total population—is more than the populations of Bangladesh, Nepal, and Pakistan combined.

Beyond absolute numbers, explained in part by population size, India also has the highest prevalence of VAD in South Asia. Fifty-seven percent of India's children are estimated to have subclinical VAD—which translates to about 3.54 crore (35.4 million) children under age 6 (Gragnolati, Shekar et al. 2005). And it is estimated that VAD contributes to the deaths of roughly 3,33,000 children in India each year (Gragnolati, Shekar et al. 2005).

The positive news is that clinical VAD has generally declined in India over the past 30 years, as indicated by a decreased prevalence of Bitot's spots among young children in rural areas (Figure 1-4). Reports suggest that prior to the 1980s, prevalence of Bitot's spots was at least 4 percent (the WHO cutoff indicating a public health problem is 0.5 percent); since then, levels have declined dramatically. A NNMB assessment showed improvements in vitamin A status between the mid-1970s and the mid-1990s (Vijayaraghavan, Balakrishna et al. 2000). However, the same study also showed that only 11 percent of the surveyed population had adequate intake of vitamin A, and 50 to 70 percent had intakes less than 30 percent of the reference daily intake (the highest amount of a nutrient recommended for an adult age group) as recently as the 1990s (see Vitamin A Sources and Daily Requirements, below). Thus, even though levels of VAD have fallen since the 1980s, it remains a persistent problem (Toteja and Singh 2004), and more recent data suggest a possible resurgence (Mason, Bailes et al. 2005).

Figure 1-4. Prevalence of Bitot's Spots among Preschool Children

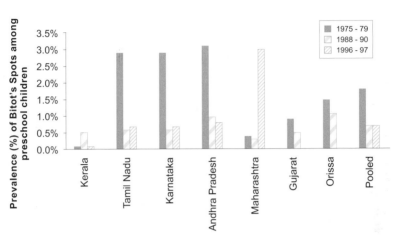

Source: NNMB 1999
Note: Pooled data refer only to states listed

Variations by State

As Figure 1-4 shows, the severity of VAD varies across states, and it has also changed considerably within states over time. The prevalence of Bitot's spots in children aged 1 to 6 in 20 states ranges from a low of 0.02 percent in Himachal Pradesh to a high of 3.94 percent in Uttar Pradesh, with 11 states above the WHO 0.5 percent indicator (Figure 1-5). Findings from several surveys show that as many as 81 percent of children in Gujarat and 80 percent in Andhra Pradesh have low serum retinol levels, indicating subclinical VAD (Table 1-1).

Despite the significant problem that VAD represents, Indian data are sparse. Most surveys have had limited geographic scope, and they do not all use the same methodology. Thus, the numbers cannot be considered definitive, but they do indicate the severity of the problem and identify the states where the problem may be greatest. Since VAD is typically a disease that especially afflicts the poor, it tends to be concentrated in states and localities with high concentrations of poor people. However, as noted

14

above, other factors, including level of other diseases and level of education of women, contribute to and increase the variation among states.

Figure 1-5. Prevalence of Bitot's Spots among Children in 17 Indian States

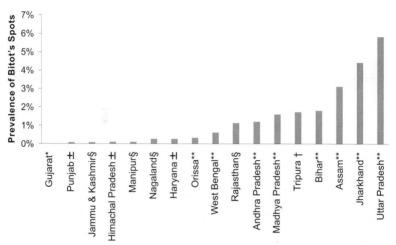

Sources: *NNMB 2002; **NNMB 2003a; §Toteja, Singh et al. 2001; ±NIN 2001; †Chakravarty and Ghosh 2000

Table 1-1. Children with Low Serum Retinol (<0.7 µmol/L)

State	Year	Percentage
Tamil Nadu	1995	16.9%
Andhra Pradesh	1989	80.0%
Delhi	1997	26.3%
Uttar Pradesh	2000	59.7%
Mahrashtra	1996	77.0%
Gujarat	1986	81.0%

Source: Toteja and Singh 2004
Note: The International Vitamin A Consultative Group and others consider levels below 0.7 µmol/L a VAD indicator.

Very few studies have been undertaken in India measuring blood levels of serum retinol because diagnosing clinical VAD through corneal evaluations and other methods is less expensive and comparatively easy. This may explain the low number of serum retinol studies and the wide disparities in some cases between the estimated levels of VAD and the recorded levels of Bitot's spots. One might expect that high levels of VAD would result in higher levels of Bitot's spots and other forms of xerophthalmia, but early studies of VAD in Denmark found that progressive VAD manifests itself as growth retardation accompanied by reduced resistance to infection, prior to the appearance of ocular problems due to xerophthalmia (Sommer and West 1996).

Other Prisms: Age, Gender, Income, Urban versus Rural

An examination of data disaggregated by such characteristics as gender, age, per capita income, and urban or rural residence further shows the impact of VAD in India.

In most age groups, a slightly higher percentage of females are affected. As described more fully below (see Consumption in India, below), the NNMB's 2000 survey, disaggregated by gender for individuals aged 10 and older, showed that more females than males consumed less than 30 percent of the reference daily intake of vitamin A, except for ages 13 through 15 (NNMB 2000). The percentages of children who consumed less than 30 percent of the recommended amounts of vitamin A were extremely high: 69.8 percent for ages 1 to 3; 60.8 percent for ages 4 to 6; and 70.8 percent for ages 7 to 9. (Sex-disaggregated data were not reported for ages below 10.) Given what is known about the importance of vitamin A for growth and resistance to disease, the high proportion of young children with such low vitamin A intake is a critical health issue with far-reaching implications.

Households with the lowest income per capita typically consume the least amounts of vitamin A, as well as other essential micronutrients, such as iron, iodine, and zinc. The 2003 NNMB survey, for instance, found higher incidences of Bitot's spots among households belonging to a Scheduled Caste or Scheduled Tribe, those engaged in agricultural labor, those with an illiterate adult female, and those without a sanitary latrine (NNMB 2003b). Other studies have also documented large divides in childhood mortality based on caste and gender (Subramanian, Nandy et al. 2006) and on the educational level of the mother (Gopalan 1999).

About 5 percent of pregnant women in India have subclinical VAD, and almost 12 percent reported that they suffered from night blindness during their most recent pregnancy (West Jr. 2002). Though rates for night blindness can vary dramatically from state to state—from as low as 0.8 percent to as high as 23.9 percent (Toteja and Singh 2004)—these parallel the highest figures in the region (Figure 1-6) and are higher than in many other regions of the world.

Figure 1-6. Prevalence of Maternal Subclinical VAD and Night Blindness, by Region and Selected Countries of South Asia

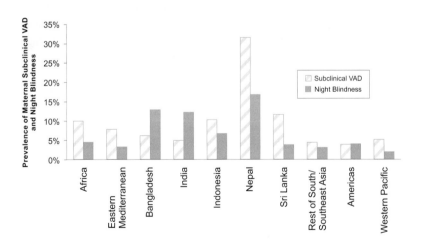

Source: West Jr. 2002

VAD is a serious problem among urban and rural Indians, with both groups consuming less than 60 percent of the average recommended daily allowance (RDA) (see below). This is most pronounced at the lowest income levels. Interestingly, despite higher overall levels of vitamin A intake by urban Indians, the rural poor consume more vitamin A than their urban counterparts at the lowest level of income (Figure 1-7). Studies over the years have confirmed the fact that urban slum dwellers have significantly high levels of malnutrition. (See Ghosh and Shah 2004 for a review of studies of urban slum children's nutritional status.) With India's urban population growing at more than twice that of the rural areas—by 2020, 40 percent of the population is expected to live in urban areas (www. unhabitat.org), about one-third of whom are expected to live in slums—the need to ensure better nutrition for the urban poor, including vitamin A and other micronutrients, will only increase.

Figure 1-7. Average Dietary Intake of Vitamin A across Urban and Rural Areas of India

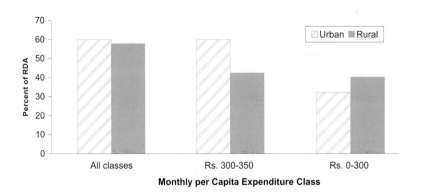

Source: Micronutrient Initiative 2005

The Health and Economic Impacts of Insufficient Vitamin A

Several factors, often acting together, cause VAD: low dietary intake, as described above, exacerbated by malabsorption and increased excretion associated with common illnesses (WHO 2002). However, the major cause of VAD—a lack of dietary intake of vitamin A—is generally related to total caloric intake. That is, the more calories people eat, the more likely they are to consume an adequate amount of vitamin A. In general, higher income leads to higher intake of nutrients such as protein (as when households switch from grains to meat and other animal products), iron, fat, and other micronutrients, which have significant direct effects on people's health as well as on their absorption of vitamin A (Jalal, Nesheim et al. 1998; Takyi 1999; Dijkhuizen, Wieringa et al. 2004). Although the link between income and caloric intake is especially strong at low income levels, there is also evidence that increased income may lead to larger household sizes and, thus, no increase in the quality or quantity of each household member's food consumption (Osmani 1997).

Infections are another cause of VAD. Repeated infections may hamper the body's utilization of calories: parasitic infections may divert nutrients for their own purposes, diarrheal diseases may increase the waste of calories, and other diseases may reduce a person's appetite (Osmani 1997). Thus, increasing caloric intake without accounting for diseases may have little effect on nutritional status. This implies that nutritional interventions alone are not enough to address VAD; prevention of infection and access to treatment are also necessary.

Health Impacts

Besides being the leading source of preventable blindness in developing countries, VAD has been shown to result in increased mortality, impaired growth, and vulnerability to infection (Sommer 1997). By compromising the immune system, VAD makes people, especially children, more susceptible to diseases that can become more serious or fatal than would otherwise be likely (Rice, West Jr. et al. 2004).

VAD contributes to the severity of the top four causes of child mortality in developing countries: lower respiratory infections, diarrheal diseases, malaria, and measles (WHO 2003). According to Rice, West Jr., et al. (2004), approximately 20 to 24 percent of child mortality from measles, diarrhea, and malaria, as well as 20 percent of all-cause maternal mortality, can be attributed to VAD. In addition, VAD is estimated to contribute to 16 percent of the global burden of disease caused by malaria and to a significant percentage of acute respiratory infections (WHO 2003; Caulfield, Richard et al. 2004). Adequate amounts of vitamin A can reduce the incidence of severe episodes of diarrhea (Bhandari, Bhan et al. 1994; Sempertegui, Estrella et al. 1999; Villamor, Mbise et al. 2002) and measles (Ramakrishnan and Martorell 1998; D'Souza and D'Souza 2002), as well as aid in growth promotion. In addition, vitamin A has been shown to play a role in reducing the most severe effects of HIV and malaria in children (Villamor, Mbise et al. 2002). As discussed above, however, this represents only the potentially avertable mortality; other factors, such as diet or initial serum levels, significantly alter the likelihood of success.

Worldwide, almost 2.1 crore (21 million) disability-adjusted life years (DALYs)[3] are estimated to be lost by children from birth through age 4 because of VAD, about 25 percent (47.6 lakh or 4.76 million DALYs) of which are in South Asia (Rice, West Jr. et al. 2004). In India, VAD results in an estimated loss of 4.04–23 lakh (4,04,000 to 2.3 million) DALYs annually (Gragnolati, Shekar et al. 2005; Stein, Sachdev et al. 2006), and as noted earlier, more than 3,30,000 Indian children under age 6 die each year because of VAD.

Economic Impacts

Three economic arguments are commonly put forward to justify investing in nutrition: (1) improving nutrition increases productivity and economic growth; (2) not addressing malnutrition has high costs in terms of higher health spending as well as lost gross domestic product (GDP); and (3) returns from programs for improving nutrition far outweigh their costs (World Bank 2005).

Based on estimates by the World Bank, improving a person's

nutritional status can result in a growth in individual lifetime earnings of at least 10 percent. Taken collectively, a population's nutritional status can make a difference of 2 to 3 percent in a country's GDP (World Bank 2005). Vitamin A is a central component of nutrition, and thus improved vitamin A status of a population could increase a country's GDP. Estimates suggest that about 5 percent of GDP in South Asia is lost each year because of deficiencies in the intakes of just three nutrients: iron, vitamin A, and iodine (World Bank 1994). Nutrition and economic growth have also been shown to be mutually reinforcing: better nutrition leads to increased human capital and labor productivity through improved health and education, which in turn results in improved household and national welfare and in overall economic growth. To complete the circle, greater economic growth (usually measured in terms of per capita GDP) results in better nutrition, principally through increased public and private spending on health, education, and food consumption (FAO 2001).

VAD also results in significant outlays for health services, in that many cases of preventable illnesses strain health systems. Conversely, strategies that reduce VAD can lower the demand for these services, and they have been shown to be cost-effective. For example, an examination of the Nepal National Vitamin A Program, which provides vitamin A supplementation, found that the impact on the incidence and severity of diarrheal disease and measles reduced the need for Ministry of Health services, saving the government approximately Rs. 6 crore (US$1.5 million annually). With an annual cost of only Rs. 67.2 lakh (US$167,000), or about Rs. 50 (US$1.25) per participant, the program has net cost savings of around Rs. 4.4 crore ($1.1 million) (Fiedler 2000), or about Rs. 13,161 (US$327) per averted death. Other studies reported Rs. 6,560 and 10,988 (US$163 and $275) per death averted in Zambia and Ghana, respectively (MOST 2004a, 2004b)[4].

In India, in addition to the physical and psychosocial toll on individuals and families, VAD has a measurable effect on the economy. According to the Micronutrient Initiative (2005), micronutrient deficiencies cost India 1 percent of its GDP. VAD is estimated to cost India Rs. 1,608 crore (US$0.4 billion) annually in lost GDP, and total micronutrient deficiencies, including VAD, may cost India Rs. 10,000 crore (US$2.5 billion) annually.

Vitamin A Sources and Daily Requirements

Vitamin A can be consumed as retinol in animal foods, such as meat, dairy products, eggs and breast milk, or as carotenoids (principally beta-carotene) in many fruits and vegetables, such as dark green leafy vegetables, mangoes, and squash. Preformed vitamin A is abundant in the animal-derived foods; provitamin A carotenoids (such as beta-carotene) are abundant in dark-colored fruits and vegetables, as well as oily fruits and some edible oils.

Absorption of preformed vitamin A and provitamin A occurs in the small intestine, which converts them to retinol and various byproducts. Preformed vitamin A is much more efficiently absorbed, with approximately 70 to 90 percent converted directly into retinol (IOM 2000). This absorption continues even at high levels of intake, and excess vitamin A is stored in the liver. Provitamin A carotenoids, on the other hand, are not absorbed nearly as efficiently. Studies have suggested that in the optimal case—purified beta-carotene in oil—one needs to consume 2 μg of beta-carotene to obtain 1 μg of retinol, a ratio of 2:1 (IOM 2000). The efficiency of beta-carotene absorption from other food products is even less than that of oil. Until recently, it was believed that 6 μg of beta-carotene in food equaled 1 μg of retinol (a ratio of 6:1), but new evidence suggests that the ratio is closer to 12:1, meaning that past recommendations about the amount of fruits and vegetables needed to meet the RDA were underestimates (IOM 2000). In addition to beta-carotene, many foods contain other provitamin A carotenoids, such as alpha-carotene. However, these are absorbed even less efficiently than beta-carotene. Based on studies estimating that the vitamin A activity of non-beta-carotene carotenoids is about half that of beta-carotene, the retinol equivalent is 24 μg per gram (a ratio of 24:1) (IOM 2000).

In all cases, those are only gross representations because the bioavailability of vitamin A varies. Factors that influence the bioavailability of vitamin A from provitamin A carotenoids include an individual's fat intake, the type of food, and its preparation (see Boileau, Moore et al. 1999 for a food matrix on bioavailability). How long and in what manner foods were stored (Rodriguez-Amaya 1997), the presence of parasites in the body (Jalal, Nesheim et al. 1998), and the stores of vitamin A in the liver as opposed to serum retinol concentrations (Ribaya-Mercado, Solon et al. 2000) are also important variables. Cooking can have adverse or positive effects. For instance, steaming can denature proteins, which releases more carotenoids, but boiling, frying, or other types of cooking at higher temperatures can destroy a significant percentage of the carotenoids (Boileau, Moore et al. 1999). Light destroys the carotenoids in spinach during storage (Boileau, Moore et al. 1999) and can also reduce the level of beta-carotene in oil (Rodriguez-Amaya 1997). In addition, people who are deficient in vitamin A seem to be more efficient at processing vitamin A than those replete with the vitamin (Sommer and West 1996)[5].

Treating children with antiparasitic drugs or increasing their fat intake has been shown to be as useful in increasing serum retinol concentrations as increased consumption of beta-carotene-rich foods (Jalal, Nesheim et al. 1998). Serum retinol concentrations may not accurately assess the level of VAD, however. Recently added vitamin A most likely circulates in the blood and is not stored in the liver in people with low vitamin A status, so measuring a person's serum retinol concentration may not always be a good indicator of her long-term vitamin A status[6] (Ribaya-Mercado, Mazariegos et al. 1999; Ribaya-Mercado, Solon et al. 2000; Tanumihardjo 2004).

Some plant foods, particularly orange and yellow vegetables, such as sweet potatoes, have much higher levels of beta-carotene than green leafy vegetables and could provide significant levels of vitamin A, but they are often only seasonably available (Miller, Humphrey et al. 2002). Some oils, particularly red palm oil, are high in beta-carotene and have been shown to be useful in improving vitamin A status when added to a deficient diet (van Stuijvenberg, Dhansay et al. 2001; Zagre, Delpeuch et al. 2003). In addition, oils convert to vitamin A at much higher rates than most other vegetable sources because of their fat content (You, Parker et al. 2002). The convertibility of beta-carotene facilitated by fat makes oil a potentially valuable fortification vehicle, as will be discussed in later chapters.

It is also important to understand how children become vitamin A deficient. The deficiency in the mother results in low concentrations for supporting the fetus (which leads in part to low birth weight) and low concentrations in breast milk (which compromises the vitamin A status of the infant). Then, during the first two years of life, many Indian children do not get enough dietary intake of vitamin A because of either a paucity of food or a lack of vitamin A sources. According to one study, a typical child in the developing world without supplementation would need to receive 10 times the intake of fruits and vegetables to meet "minimally adequate" levels of vitamin A (Miller, Humphrey et al. 2002); the authors conclude that without animal products, it is virtually impossible for children to consume enough vitamin A through their diet.

Daily Requirements

The U.S. Institute of Medicine (IOM) has established RDAs for vitamin A that vary by age and, for adults, by sex (Table 1-2). These amounts are listed as µg of retinol activity equivalents (RAE), which allow a common standard across different foods. The RDAs are based on the amount needed to meet the nutrient requirement of nearly all (97 to 98 percent) healthy people of a specific age group and sex[7]. In India, the Indian Council of Medical Research sets RDAs, which are comparable in most age classes to those set by the IOM.

Table 1-2. Vitamin A RDAs in the United States and India

	U.S. RDAs (µg RAE/day)	Indian RDAs (µg RAE/day)
0–6 months	400*	350
7–12 months	500*	350
1–3 years	300	400
4–8 years	400	400 (4–6 years)
		600 (7–9 years)
9–13 years	600	600 (10–18 years)
Pregnant females	750–770	N/A
Lactating females	1200–1300	950
Other females, 14 and older	700	600
Males, 14 and older	900	600

*Adequate intake, rather than RDA, is used for children under age 1, based on recommendations from the U.S. Institute of Medicine. Adequate intake is the amount that appears to be sufficient when other measurements are not possible to obtain, given the age of the infant. It is also recommended that infants under 6 months receive all their nutrients through breast milk.

Sources: IOM 2000; ICMR 1995

A pregnant woman depletes her vitamin A stores more quickly than a nonpregnant woman, which affects both her own health and that of her fetus. A lactating woman needs almost twice as much vitamin A daily as other women to sustain herself and her infant (IOM 2000).

As noted in the previous section, many factors affect how much vitamin A is absorbed into the body, but even gross representations provide a useful basis for analyzing diet. People who rely on fruits and vegetables for their vitamin A intake will have a hard time getting sufficient amounts through normal daily food consumption. It is clear why VAD remains a serious issue in much of the developing world, where retinol sources from dairy, meat, and other animal products are less available for many people (IOM 2000).

Consumption in India

Consumption of vitamin A in India is largely insufficient to meet the RDAs at all ages, especially among females (Figure 1-8).

Figure 1-8. Mean Daily Intake of Vitamin A by Age Groups and Sex

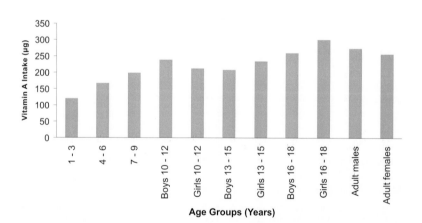

Source: Vijayaraghavan, Balakrishna et al. 2000 (Table 13)

In rural areas of India, 50 to 60 percent of women consume 30 percent or less of the recommended vitamin A daily intake (Vijayaraghavan 2006). In one study in Tamil Nadu, mothers with low micronutrient consumption– from inadequate consumption of milk, green leafy vegetables, and fruit– delivered infants of low birth weight, an important predictor of malnutrition and other health problems later in life (Rao, Yajnik et al. 2001). After birth, infants can become further vitamin A deficient if they breastfeed from mothers who are themselves vitamin A-deficient, and their condition then worsens if they are weaned onto foods with insufficient amounts of the vitamin (Miller, Humphrey et al. 2002).

The average percentages of RDA of children under age 6 are presented in Figure 1-9. The numbers reported in the figure are the average vitamin A intake for pooled boys and girls at ages 1–3 and 4–6.

Figure 1-9. Percentage of RDA of Vitamin A Consumed by Children under 6, by State

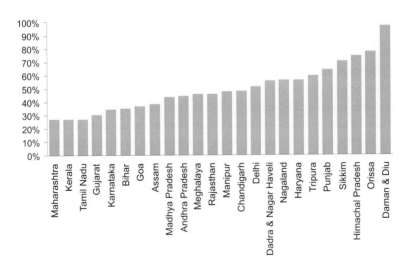

Source: Toteja and Singh 2004

Summary

Prevalence. Worldwide, vitamin A deficiency results in 12–30 lakh (1.2–3 million) childhood deaths; as many as 25.4 crore (254 million) children may have VAD disorders. In India, about 57 percent of children—more than 3.5 crore (35 million)—do not get enough vitamin A, and the problem is particularly acute among the rural and urban poor in most states. VAD leads to the deaths of 3,30,000 children in India each year. About 5 percent of pregnant women have subclinical VAD and 12 percent report night blindness during their most recent pregnancy.

Health and economic impacts. VAD can cause blindness and turn many childhood diseases in developing countries—including measles, diarrhea, and malaria—into more serious and even deadly conditions by compromising immunity. Worldwide, it is estimated that almost 2.1 crore (21 million) DALYs are lost to VAD annually. In India, the loss due to VAD is estimated at 4.04–23 lakh (4,04,000 to 2.3 million) DALYs annually, with an estimated annual impact on the economy of Rs. 1,608 crore ($0.4 billion).

Necessary intake. The U.S. Institute of Medicine and the National Institute of Nutrition in India have both set recommended amounts of vitamin A for different age groups and for men and women. Adequate vitamin A intake requires more retinol activity equivalents from vegetable sources than from animal products—in other words, far larger amounts of fruits and vegetables and their products must be consumed to derive vitamin A. In the 1990s, on average, 50 to 70 percent of Indian children consumed less than 30 percent of the recommended amounts, with the urban and rural poor at particular risk.

Notes

[1]Xerophthalmia (Greek for "dry eyes") is a medical condition in which the eye fails to produce tears because of inadequate functioning of the lacrimal glands. When xerophthalmia is due to VAD, the condition begins with night blindness and conjunctival xerosis (dryness of the eye membranes) and progresses to corneal xerosis (dryness of the cornea), and in the late stages, to keratomalacia (softening of the cornea), which can lead to permanent blindness.

[2]Clinical VAD is generally measured by incidence of night blindness, Bitot's spots, or other forms of xerophthalmia; subclinical VAD is generally measured by serum retinol levels. Many experts do not distinguish between clinical and subclinical symptoms but refer to broader VAD disorders (West Jr. 2002).

[3]DALYs are a measure of healthy life years: the sum of the present value of years of future lifetime lost through premature mortality, and the present value of years of future lifetime adjusted for the average severity of the mental or physical disability caused by a disease or injury (Rushby and Hanson 2001).

[4]The Ghana program cost Rs. 8,774–23,586 (US$218–586) based on total costs and Rs. 2,455–6,560 (US$61–163) for program-specific costs only. For Zambia, total costs were Rs. 3,622–11,068 (US$90–275), and program-specific costs were Rs. 1,408–4,306 (US$35–107). Results vary based on assumptions about the decline in mortality. Chapter 2 describes this analysis in greater detail.

[5]Recent studies among healthy, well-fed men have found significant variation in the conversion of beta-carotene into vitamin A (Hickenbottom, Follett et al. 2002), suggesting that some of the variability among people may be innate.

[6]In people with adequate intake of vitamin A, more than 90 percent of total vitamin A is found in the liver.

[7]The method of determining the RDAs for vitamins and minerals is beyond the scope of this paper but can be found in Dietary Reference Intakes (IOM 2000). The IOM based the RDA for individuals on a population-wide standard called estimated average requirements, defined as the nutrient intake level estimated to meet the needs of 50 percent of a particular population plus two standard deviations—thus encompassing about 98 percent, assuming a normal distribution. Another standard cited in some studies is the reference daily intake, which is the highest amount of a nutrient recommended for an adult age group.

CHAPTER 2

Addressing Vitamin A Deficiencies

Evidence that vitamin A deficiency is a causal factor for child mortality catalyzed efforts beginning in the 1980s to increase vitamin A intake among children, even if they did not have the eye-related problems traditionally associated with VAD. This chapter reviews the three interventions most commonly used: high-dosage supplementation, food fortification, and other food-based approaches, such as dietary diversification. We summarize how these strategies have been used and focus on attempts to assess the costs and explain the success or failure of some of the programs. This discussion may help extract lessons learned if production of biofortified mustard or other foods is used to increase vitamin A intake in India.

Supplementation

Supplementation provides high doses of vitamin A to offset poor nutrition and prevent the morbidity and mortality associated with VAD. Through large doses on a periodic basis (optimally, twice a year), supplementation aims to improve vitamin A status by building up stores of vitamin A in the liver and tissues. Supplementation is usually set up as a nationwide or regional program to administer synthetically produced, high-dosage vitamin A capsules or, as in India, an oily syrup solution to the targeted population. WHO and UNICEF recommend that supplementation be integrated into routine and supplemental immunization activities as a preventive measure in developing countries (Ching, Birmingham et al. 2000).

WHO has established recommended dosages (Table 2-1) for supplementation for young children at four- to six-month intervals and for postpartum women between the time of delivery and up to six months afterward—the period in which a mother ideally is breastfeeding her infant. Routine supplementation is not recommended for pregnant women unless they are at risk of blindness due to xerophthalmia because of potential overdosage effects on the fetus, especially early in pregnancy (see Box 2-1). Although it is recommended that infants younger than 9 months receive vitamin A through breast milk, they may be administered a 50,000-IU high-dosage supplement of vitamin A without significant risks (Sommer and West 1996).

High-dosage supplementation of vitamin A can work because, unlike many other micronutrients, the body stores excess amounts of vitamin A for future use. The body retains approximately 50 percent of a large dose, though likely less in children suffering from malnutrition and infection (Sommer and West 1996). Prophylactic vitamin A supplementation does not address the underlying causes of VAD. Rather, it is intended to prevent VAD among high-risk individuals until more adequate and sustainable dietary interventions become effective, though it has proven hard in practice to withdraw supplementation and rely only on diet (Sommer and West 1996)

Table 2-1. Potential Target Groups and Recommended Dosages in Countries with VAD

Target group	Vitamin A dose*
All mothers irrespective of their mode of infant feeding up to 6 weeks postpartum if they have not received vitamin A supplementation after delivery	2,00,000 IUs†
Infants 9–11 months	1,00,000 IUs
Children 12 months and older	2,00,000 IUs
Children 1–4 years	2,00,000 IUs

* The optimal interval between doses (administered orally) is 4 to 6 months. A dose should not be given too soon after a previous dose of vitamin A supplement: the minimum recommended interval between doses for the prevention of VAD is 1 month (the interval can be reduced to treat clinical VAD and measles cases).

† 2,00,000 IUs is equivalent to 60,000 µg RE or 209 µmol/L

Source: WHO (http://www.who.int/vaccines/en/vitamina.shtml)

Supplementation can also be used to cure serious cases of xerophthalmia. For individuals presenting with ocular symptoms, vitamin A supplementation is part of the usual standard of care. In addition, supplementation has been shown to be effective in improving health outcomes for individuals with measles, diarrheal diseases, HIV, and malnutrition (Bhandari, Bhan et al. 1994; Fawzi, Mbise et al. 2000).

Box 2-1
Toxicity of Vitamin A

Vitamin A is absorbed fairly quickly into the body and, once introduced, tends to accumulate. Vitamin A can become toxic, either acutely, following a sufficiently high dose, or chronically, after prolonged intake of small doses. Acute toxicities typically occur in the hours or days after the intake of a high dose, whereas chronic toxicities occur after weeks, months, or even years of amounts that are not acutely toxic. This latter condition, called hypervitaminosis A, has been observed in both adults and children. Symptoms include vomiting, nausea, headaches, and in rare cases, death (Hathcock, Hattan et al. 1990).

According to Sommer and West (1996), up to 4 percent of children 1 to 6 years old may experience acute, transient side effects, such as nausea, vomiting, headache, or fever, following intake of high dosages of vitamin A. No studies have been conducted on the effects of high dosages on children 6 to 12 months old, but dosages of 1,00,000 IUs are considered safe based on extrapolation backward from 1-year-olds (Sommer and West 1996). Infants younger than 6 months seem to have little trouble tolerating a single 50,000-IU oral dose of vitamin A; side effects may include a bulging fontanel, which, though not considered harmful, may affect caregivers' compliance decisions (Sommer and West 1996).

Women of childbearing age who may become pregnant are advised against taking high-dose capsules because of the risks of toxicity for their fetuses. Most warnings are based on a single large dose (~5,00,000 IUs), which can be teratogenic—capable of causing a malformation of the fetus—though repeated exposure to lesser doses can also produce similar defects (Hathcock, Hattan et al. 1990). However, no cases of teratogenicity have been reported with daily dosing in line with recommendations by the U.S. Food and Drug Administration. In addition, there have been no reports of problems in mothers given a high dose following childbirth. Recommendations to provide high-dose supplementation within the first 6 to 8 weeks after childbirth are due to the possibility of pregnancy with the return of ovulation after 8 weeks (Sommer and West Jr. 1996).

There has been at least one suspected outbreak of hypervitaminosis A in India. More than 14 children died and many more became sick in Assam following a vitamin A campaign in 2000 (Ramachandran 2001; West Jr. and Sommer 2002; Kapil 2004). Blame centered on UNICEF's introduction of larger dosing cups and the inexperience and poor training of health workers (Kapil 2004), though others dispute that vitamin A supplementation was the cause of death (West Jr. and Sommer 2002). Regardless, the media attention was a setback to supporters of supplementation. In sum, although there is a small risk associated with high-dose supplementation, expected decreases in morbidity related to xerophthalmia and mortality will likely continue to outweigh the risks until a diet rich in vitamin A can be adopted (West Jr. and Sommer 2002).

Sources: Hathcock, Hattan et al. 1990; Sommer and West Jr. 1996, West Jr. and Sommer 2002, Kapil 2004

Approximately 70 percent of children in 40 developing countries receive vitamin A supplementation at least once per year, most often with international donor support. Based on 2002–2003 figures, however, only 10 countries of those identified as needing it reached at least 70 percent of their children with the recommended two dosages per year: Burkina Faso, Ghana, Mauritania, Mongolia, Myanmar, North Korea, Niger, Oman, Pakistan, Philippines, Sierra Leone, Sudan, and Tanzania (UNICEF 2004).

Supplementation often occurs on National Immunization Days, well-promoted campaigns that provide children with polio and other immunizations. It is also carried out as part of a micronutrient or child health day (usually a well-publicized special event to reach a large number of children at one time) or as part of routine care (Ching, Birmingham et al. 2000).

Although different in their delivery mechanisms, programs in Ghana, Nepal, and Zambia share some common features that have made them successful, including clearly defined program goals, client-focused delivery mechanisms, and community support (Houston 2003).[1] In Ghana, health districts experimented with ways to promote the program, such as piggybacking on National Immunization Days and delivering supplements through schools. After evaluation, it was found that districts that used a community outreach program along with house-to-house visits had the best success. Within three years of beginning supplementation, coverage extended to nearly 100 percent of Ghana's young children. In Nepal, community health volunteers became the primary means of delivering the supplements as part of their broader health mandate, through a nongovernmental organization (NGO) charged by the Ministry of Health to implement the program (see Box 2-2). By 2001, almost every district in the country had at least 80 percent coverage in its supplementation program, up from less than 40 percent of districts covered in 1997. In Zambia, supplementation was initiated through National Immunization Days but later broadened to a program called Child Health Week, which included several preventive services for children. Supplementation coverage grew from about 30 percent in 1997 to more than 80 percent in 2001.

It is also important to weigh costs against the number of children reached. Across the three countries, the average cost per child dosed twice a year was Rs. 16 (US$0.40) if only program-specific costs were considered, and Rs. 46 (US$1.15) if personnel and capital costs were also included. Program-specific costs, including capsules, supplies, training, and social mobilization activities, represented an average of 37 percent of the total cost of supplementation in the three countries; personnel costs, such as health workers and others, constituted 48 percent of total costs; and capital costs, such as vehicles, office equipment, and other assets, represented 15 percent of total costs (MOST 2004c).

Box 2-2
Supplementation Case Study: Nepal's National Vitamin A Program

Through the Nepal National Vitamin A Program, children aged 6 months to 5 years receive high-dose vitamin A capsules twice a year. The program began in 1993 in eight districts and has since expanded nationwide. It is based on tapping into an existing cadre of female community health volunteers to distribute vitamin A capsules as part of a broader health program. The program is considered highly successful, not only because it has increased vitamin A, intake but also because it empowers and involves the volunteers in their communities. An NGO called the Technical Advisory Group assists the Ministry of Health in implementing the program; it trains the volunteer workers, monitors and supervises their activities, and provides most of the information, education, and communication to promote the program.

The total cost of the program is about Rs. 6.85 crore ($1.7 million) per year. It is estimated to decrease child mortality in Nepal by 25 to 30 percent at a cost of Rs. 13,165 (US$327) per averted death and Rs. 50 (US$1.25) to deliver two capsules to each child (Fiedler 2000). The capsules themselves represent only a tiny percentage of the cost, with promotion of the program to the public, training, and administrative costs making up most of the rest. The female community health volunteers are not compensated, but they do receive supplies and a relatively generous per diem to attend training courses.

In his analysis of the Nepal National Vitamin A Program, Fiedler (2000) considered its sustainability (it relies heavily on international donor support) and its applicability to other countries. While not advocating this program as a prototype, he identified several replicable features, particularly the training for volunteers.

Sources: Fiedler 2000; Houston 2003

Researchers who have attempted to quantify costs and cost-effectiveness of supplementation programs in other countries report a wide range of costs and cost per death averted. Depending on the study, the benefit-cost ratio has ranged from 4:1 to more than 140:1 (Behrman, Alderman et al. 2004). Even at the lowest benefit-cost ratio, 4:1, UNICEF and the World Bank consider supplementation one of the most cost-effective child survival interventions available (World Bank 1993; UNICEF 2006).

Ching, Birmingham et al. (2000) used a worldwide incremental cost of Rs. 4 (US$0.10) per child per dosage when a supplement was administered as part of an already scheduled National Immunization Day and Rs.17 (US$0.43) when administered as a stand-alone program—doubling these amounts to cover the recommended two dosages per year. Incremental costs comprised the cost of the capsule plus additional costs of training, logistics, and supplies. The stand-alone costs were estimated on the basis of WHO polio campaign cost data. Using these cost figures and estimates that supplements averted 1.69 lakh (169,000) child deaths in 1998 and 2.42 lakh (242,000) child deaths in 1999, they determined that the incremental cost per death averted was Rs. 2,895 (US$72) in 1998 (the range was Rs. 1,447–5,711, or US$36–142) and Rs. 2,574 (US $64) in 1999 (the range was Rs. 1,287–5,067, or US$32–126). The average cost per death averted was Rs. 12,468 (US$310) in 1998 (the range was Rs. 6314–24,493, or US$157–609) and Rs. 11,100 (US$276) in 1999 (the range was Rs. 5,590–21,718, or US$139–540).[2]

The Philippines' National Vitamin A Supplementation Program is another long-standing, extensive program. One analysis of its costs found that variables such as personnel and transportation expenses greatly influenced the costs in each barangay, or district (Fiedler, Dado et al. 2000). At the time of the analysis, the Philippine program reached 88 percent of children aged 1 through 6 twice a year—once during a National Immunization Day and once during a separate Micronutrient Day, although coverage had slipped from a high of 93 percent when the program began in 1993. This program is very labor intensive: the number of health workers, municipal officials, community volunteers, and others involved means that about 1.5 percent of the entire population—or more than 10 lakh (1 million) people—were involved in the program in one way or another at the time of the study. As discussed below, the costs are such that the authors suggest considering fortification as a complementary strategy to supplementation.

As important a contribution as supplementation has made, it is not a panacea. Even in the countries with relative success stories, large percentages of children still had subclinical VAD, according to UNICEF data: 66 percent in Zambia, 60 percent in Ghana, and 33 percent in Nepal (UNICEF/Micronutrient Initiative 2004). One can only assume that the situation would otherwise have been worse, yet this gap points to the need for additional interventions. And National Immunization Days, which have been an effective and efficient means to deliver vitamin A supplements in many countries, are declining in number—an ironic tribute to the success of the global polio program. As the polio campaign winds down and these immunization days are discontinued, supplementation costs may rise and programs may be more difficult to sustain, thus resulting in lower vitamin A coverage. For this reason, fortification and dietary diversification, discussed more fully below, may represent more sustainable, long-term solutions to VAD.

Supplementation in India

India launched one of the first supplementation programs in the world in 1970. Known as the National Prophylaxis Programme for the Prevention of Nutritional Blindness, it was designed to address the ocular consequences of VAD; the mortality and morbidity implications of VAD were not clearly understood at that time. It began with doses to children from ages 1 to 5 but was refined over the years to target children from 6 months to 3 years through the Reproductive and Child Health program of the Ministry of Health and Family Welfare (Reddy 2002b).

Nutrient kits, which include vitamin A supplements, are also distributed through government-run health subcenters, each of which is intended to provide coverage for 5,000 people (3,000 in tribal, hilly, or inaccessible areas) (Lakshman, pers. comm.). In practice, each center serves around 6,000 to 7,000 people, with gaps between need and distribution of the nutrient kits; large sections of the population have little or no access to the interventions. As further explored in Chapter 4, functioning subcenters have a significant effect on supplementation costs and cost-effectiveness.

Coverage of children in India is fairly low. In 2000, it was estimated that only about 31 percent of children aged 9 to 12 months received vitamin A prophylaxis (see Table 2-2), usually given with vaccinations (Vijayaraghavan 2006); thus, many were unlikely to get a second dose, and older children were unlikely to get a first dose. Coverage numbers after 2000 are likely to be similar or worse because of the cases of hypervitaminosis A and subsequent scare in Assam in 2001 (see Box 2-1 and below). A more recent survey of 2,681 children in eight states (Andhra Pradesh, Karnataka, Kerala, Madhya Pradesh, Maharashtra, Orissa, Tamil Nadu, and West Bengal) found a higher overall rate of coverage, 57.7 percent (see Table 2-3), but the survey was small and looked only at rural communities.

Table 2-2. Percentage of Children Aged 12–23 Months Who Received Vitamin A Prophylaxis at 9–12 Months

State	Rural	Urban	Total
India, total	29.2	38.6	31.4
Andaman and Nicobar Islands*	—	—	80.7
Andhra Pradesh	33.5	34.2	33.7
Arunachal Pradesh	—	—	31.3
Assam	19.7	47.2	22
Bihar	9.3	19.5	10.6
Chandigarh*	—	—	64.1
Dadra and Nagar Haveli*	—	—	69.4
Daman and Diu*	—	—	59
Delhi	52.7	44.7	45.8
Goa	88.2	76.3	82
Gujarat	44.2	49.6	45.8
Haryana	35.7	49.6	39
Himachal Pradesh	68.8	72.4	69.2
Jammu and Kashmir	43.5	65.7	47.8
Karnataka	57.9	52.9	56.3
Kerala	69.7	58.2	66.2

Lakshadweep*	—	—	81
Madhya Pradesh	28.1	30.5	28.7
Maharashtra	57.8	46	52.9
Manipur	43.9	57	47.5
Meghalaya	—	—	37.4
Mizoram	44	51.3	48.7
Nagaland	—	—	29.7
Orissa	39.4	54.8	41.6
Pondicherry*	—	—	66.7
Punjab	43.2	58.6	47.5
Rajasthan	23.6	43.3	27.6
Sikkim	—	—	45
Tamil Nadu	42.3	42.2	42.3
Tripura	—	—	29.1
Uttar Pradesh	9.2	11	9.5
West Bengal	53.6	60.8	54.9

Source: Multiple Indicator Cluster Survey (MICS)2001
*Note: *Union territories*

Table 2-3. Rural Communities' Receipt of High-Dose Vitamin A, by State

	Percentage of communities receiving high dose	Percentage change from 2000 (MICS* 2001)
Kerala	43.9	−24
Tamil Nadu	63	49
Karnataka	56.5	−2
Andhra Pradesh	50.7	51
Maharashtra	52.4	−9
Madhya Pradesh	52.6	47
Orissa	80	103
West Bengal	51.9	−3
Pooled	57.7	

* Multiple Indicator Cluster Survey
Source: NNMB 2003b

In the 2003 NNMB survey, most mothers whose children received a supplement knew that it was beneficial (60.6 percent overall, ranging from a low of 38.5 percent in Madhya Pradesh to a high of 93.1 percent in Karnataka), with "improved health" as the most commonly cited benefit (NNMB 2003b). Most of the mothers whose children did not receive a supplement said that the supplements were not offered to their children (52 percent) or they were not aware of the program (34.2 percent). Very few said that they did not take their children for supplementation because of inconvenience (5.6 percent) or fear of side effects (1.1 percent).

It is interesting to note that in Orissa, which had relatively high coverage, vitamin A was administered as part of an integrated program (Vijayaraghavan 2006) rather than as a stand-alone event. Almost one-third of the children received their supplements at an Anganwadi center, a facility affiliated with the ICDS program, which provides health services, education, and supplementary nutrition for preschool children and their mothers (Box 2-3). Yet another study had conflicting findings on the role of Anganwadi centers: in looking at villages in Kerala, Maharashtra, Rajasthan, and Uttar Pradesh that did and did not have these facilities, children were more likely to receive supplementation if their village had an Anganwadi center only in Maharashtra and Uttar Pradesh, and even there, the numbers were not adequate (Gragnolati, Shekar et al. 2005).

Box 2-3
India's Integrated Child Development Services

The ICDS program was started in 1975 by the Government of India with help from UNICEF. ICDS aims to increase child development, which is hindered by poverty, poor environmental sanitation, disease, inadequate access to health care, and poor or inappropriate child care. The ICDS approach is to introduce a package of different services including supplementary nutrition, immunization, childcare, and basic health services to children younger than 6 years old and their mothers. To meet this mission, ICDS establishes centers in mainly rural villages that are staffed by an Anganwadi worker. These workers provide immunizations, perform health checkups, and educate children and mothers about health and nutrition.

Studies have shown that the ICDS program has done little to increase child nutrition or ameliorate the problems of malnutrition, such as stunting and wasting, largely because Anganwadi workers have inadequate training, supervision, and support. In addition, services are targeted mainly at children aged 4 to 6, which is past the optimal window for influencing growth. Another major issue is that priority sites are not the poorest villages but the richest, partly because of political influence and partly because poor villages cannot support these centers. The result is that the poorest states have the worst coverage and the least allocated resources. Given all these problems, it has been hard to show that ICDS has had any measurable effect. Despite the significant human and economic costs associated with micronutrient deficiencies in general and VAD in particular, no formal cost-effectiveness studies of ICDS have been conducted, but it is not regarded as very cost-effective in reaching vulnerable populations (Horton 1999). In 2001, India's Supreme Court directed states to "universalize" ICDS to cover more communities. This may help improve efforts to increase vitamin A intake.

Sources: Horton 1999; Gupta, Lokshin et al. 2005; Lakshman 2006

The supplementation program in India uses syrup, rather than capsules, as in other countries. This approach may result in less coverage, since syrup is more expensive (Rs. 1.29 per dose of syrup compared with Rs. 0.99 for a capsule in a plastic jar) and harder to handle and distribute efficiently (Anand, Sankar et al. 2004). Vinodini Reddy, former director of the National Institute of Nutrition, has cited costs of Rs. 3.20 (about US$0.07) per child per year for universal supplementation but notes that a strategy to target only the districts where VAD is a public health problem would be more cost-effective (Reddy 2002b).

Supplementation is not universally supported in India. The 2000 National Consultation on the Benefits and Safety of Vitamin A Administration concluded that "available data are not robust enough to persuade us to recommend a policy of vitamin A supplementation for the purpose of mortality reduction in children" (National Consultation 2001), although the panel did not recommend ending the program. Rather, a "holistic approach" to combat nutritional deficiencies was recommended: "for sustainable elimination of VAD, production and consumption of vitamin A rich foods must be strongly promoted in the community, particularly among pregnant and lactating women and children." The Indian Academy of Pediatrics also recommended against combining vitamin A supplementation with polio immunization for three reasons: "(1) there is unambiguous evidence of appreciable secular decline in clinical vitamin A deficiency in under-five children in the country; (2) recent data indicates that vitamin A supplementation in infancy does not have any beneficial effect on growth, morbidity and mortality; (3) it was felt that linking vitamin A to the pulse polio program is inappropriate; the routine program should not be destabilized except under exceptional circumstances" (IAP 2002). In October 2005, the Indian Academy of Pediatrics endorsed supplementation for children aged 9 months to 3 years, but not for older children unless they had been diagnosed with severe protein energy malnutrition, severe malnourishment, or measles (IAP 2005).

Another setback for supplementation supporters, referred to in Box 2-1, was the deaths of at least 14 children and the illness of hundreds more who had received 25,000 IUs of vitamin A during a large-scale campaign in Assam in 2001 (Ramachandran 2001; West Jr. and Sommer 2002; Kapil 2004). A government investigation revealed that the overdoses occurred because cups were used rather than the smaller-dose spoons. The number of children stricken was tiny compared with the total number receiving the supplements (estimated at 28 lakh, or 2.8 million), and it is possible that some of the deaths occurred from other causes. Nonetheless, the fallout, in terms of heightened media coverage, public concern, and calls to end the focus on single-nutrient campaigns, was considerable.

Fortification

Fortification is a process in which one or more nutrients are added to commonly consumed foods, boosting the levels naturally present. Fortification contrasts with enrichment, which is the replacement of nutrients normally found in a food that are lost during food processing. The main aim of vitamin A fortification is to correct the vitamin deficiency of susceptible populations by adding a sufficient amount of vitamin A, but not enough to risk overdosing those who consume large amounts of the product. As with any fortificant, the vitamin A should not alter the taste, texture, or smell of the product, and potency should remain high under usual conditions of processing, transport, storage, and cooking.

Fortification offers an opportunity to improve micronutrient status without changing food habits, since the same foods in the same amounts, albeit fortified, are consumed (Sommer and West 1996). In addition to expanding vitamin A coverage to children and lactating women not reached by supplements, fortified food can also raise the intake by other women of childbearing age and by school-age children, who are typically not targets of supplementation programs, as well as by pregnant women who are not supposed to take supplements except under specific circumstances (Dary and Mora 2002). In addition, unlike supplementation, food fortification can bypass often-overburdened health systems.

Fortification Worldwide

Fortification has been used for more than 80 years. In the United States, fortification began in the 1920s with iodine-fortified salt and in the 1930s with vitamin D-fortified milk. In another early application, margarine was fortified with vitamin A in Denmark in the 1920s when it was found that switching to margarine from butter led to increased incidences of night blindness (Dary and Mora 2002). Vitamin A-fortified foods in developing countries today include sugar in Central America, as well as more limited fortification of flour, margarine, rice, oil, and monosodium glutamate (MSG) in various countries (Caulfield, Richard et al. 2006).

Some nutrition experts contend that fortification's full potential to increase consumption has not been tapped in developing countries (ACC/SCN 2000), and, in fact, fortification must meet several conditions to be effective (Dary and Mora 2002). The food must be consumed regularly and produced in a few centralized sites. Fortification must not affect the look or taste of the food and should provide at least 15 percent of RDA. Most challenging to developing countries, fortification must be regulated, monitored, and marketed effectively. In addition, fortification must be combined with other strategies, particularly supplementation, to reach those not covered by fortification alone, such as infants and small children. These conditions limit its applicability in many places where the population would benefit from increased vitamin A.

Data on consumption patterns of the food under consideration for fortification are essential to determine how much vitamin A (or other micronutrient) can be safely added and to ensure that the target population consumes the food in sufficient quantity to benefit (Roche/OMNI/USAID 1997) without being at risk from overdosing. Other necessary information includes knowledge about marketing and distribution of the food under consideration, and economic and technical feasibility. Thus, sugar was selected as a vehicle for fortification in Central America because, among other reasons, it is centrally produced, purchased in the marketplace, and widely consumed (see Box 2-4). Likewise, in the Philippines, wheat flour was selected over sugar and cooking oil because there are only 12 flour millers nationwide, the millers already enriched their products and expressed willingness to undertake fortification, and all but one already had the necessary quality-assurance equipment (Fiedler, Dado et al. 2000).

Edible oils are potentially ideal candidates for vitamin A fortification, since, as noted in Chapter 1, vitamin A is fat-soluble and thus more easily absorbed by the body when in oil. Methods for fortifying oils with vitamin A are well established, fairly simple, and easy to implement at low cost (Favaro, Ferreira et al. 1991; Bagriansky and Ranum 1998; Dary and Mora 2002). In fact, the U.S. Food Aid Program, Canadian International Development Agency, and United Nations World Food Programme provide vitamin A-fortified vegetable oil in their food assistance programs. Nevertheless, oils have not been widely fortified (Dary and Mora 2002). The main problem is that in many countries, including India, cooking oils are typically manufactured by many small processors, which would make a policy of mandatory fortification difficult to implement.

As with supplementation, the costs and cost-effectiveness of fortification vary based on the country, food to be fortified, ancillary costs, and other factors. Dary and Mora (2002) compiled data on fortification costs to provide 180 µg RAEs through four vehicles: oil or margarine, cereal flours, sugar, and MSG (see Table 2-4). In their analysis, oil or margarine carries by far the lowest per capita cost, Rs. 0.30 (US$0.008), because marginal costs are increased far less than with the other foods, possibly because vitamin A absorption is easiest from oil and the amount needed is far less than in dry products. In addition, it is easier to add the vitamin A to oil and it is far more stable, again meaning less is needed to achieve the same gain. They did, however, identify as a constraint to any fortification efforts the reluctance of producers to add costs, out of concern that their products would be more expensive and thus less competitive compared with nonfortified equivalents.[3] This concern reinforces the importance of laws or regulations that set and enforce nutritional standards so that all producers are operating on a level playing field. Even supposedly mandatory programs (Table 2-5) often fall short in practice because of weak monitoring and enforcement.

Table 2-4. Comparative Costs to Supply 180 µg of Retinol Equivalent (i.e., 30% Recommended Daily Intake)

Food matrix	Typical consumption g/day	Level[1] at households mg/kg	Level at stores[2] mg/kg	Overage or production[3] (percentage)	Cost in Rs./MT (US$/MT)	Percentage of purchasing price	Annual cost per person in Rs. (US$)
Oil or margarine	15	12	15	20	75 (1.87)	0.37	.32 (0.008)
Cereal flours	200	1	1.25	40	50 (1.25)	0.26	3.7 (0.091)
Sugar	50	3.5	4.5	100	268 (6.65)	1.39	4.9 (0.121)
MSG	0.25	720	900	100	50,969 (1266)[4]	25.32	4.6 (0.116)

1 Level = dietary goal (µg of retinol equivalent)/consumption pattern (g/day)
2 Assuming 25% additional amount to compensate for any losses
3 Theoretical estimate based on reported stability information and length of product marketing life
4 Assuming that MSG costs Rs. 200/kg (US$5/kg)

Source: Dary and Mora 2002 (Table 2)

Table 2-5. Mandatory Food Fortification Programs in 26 Countries

Country	Food vehicle(s)	Nutrient
Bolivia	Wheat flour	Thiamine, riboflavin, niacin, folic acid, iron
Brazil	Dried skimmed milk for complementary food programs	Vitamins A and D
Chile	Wheat flour	Thiamine, riboflavin, niacin, folic acid, iron
	Pasta	Thiamine, riboflavin, niacin, iron
	Margarine	Vitamins A and D
Colombia	Wheat flour	Thiamine, riboflavin, niacin, folic acid, iron
	Margarine	Vitamins A and D
Costa Rica	Wheat flour	Thiamine, riboflavin, niacin, folic acid, iron
	Sugar	Vitamin A
Dominican Republic	Wheat flour	Thiamine, riboflavin, niacin, folic acid, iron
Ecuador	Wheat flour	Thiamine, riboflavin, niacin, folic acid, iron
	Margarine	Vitamins A and D
El Salvador	Wheat flour	Thiamine, riboflavin, niacin, folic acid, iron
	Margarine, sugar	Vitamin A

Guatemala	Wheat flour	Thiamine, riboflavin, niacin, folic acid, iron, calcium
	Pasta	Thiamine, riboflavin, niacin, iron
	Skimmed milk	Vitamins A and D
	Margarine, sugar	Vitamin A
Honduras	Wheat flour	Thiamine, riboflavin, niacin, folic acid, iron
	Milk, margarine	Vitamins A and D
	Sugar	Vitamin A
Mexico	Sterilized low-fat milk, pasteurized low-fat milk, evaporated whole and low-fat milk, margarine or spreads	Vitamins A and D
Nicaragua	Wheat flour	Thiamine, riboflavin, niacin, folic acid, iron
	Sugar	Vitamin A
Panama	Wheat flour	Thiamine, riboflavin, niacin, folic acid, iron
	Sugar	Vitamin A
Paraguay	Wheat flour	Thiamine, riboflavin, niacin, folic acid, iron
Peru	Wheat flour	Iron
	Margarine	Vitamins A and D
Venezuela	Wheat flour	Thiamine, riboflavin, niacin, iron
	Precooked maize flour	Thiamine, riboflavin, niacin, vitamin A, iron
	Dried milk powder	Vitamins A and D
Nigeria	Enriched flour	Thiamine, riboflavin, niacin, iron, calcium
South Africa	Enriched maize meal	Riboflavin, niacin
	Margarine	Vitamins A and D
Zambia	Sugar	Vitamin A
India	Vanaspati, margarine	Vitamin A
Indonesia	Wheat flour	Thiamine, riboflavin, iron, zinc
	Margarine	Vitamins A and D
Malaysia	Evaporated milk, condensed milk, filled milk	Vitamin A
	Table margarine	Vitamins A and D
Pakistan	Oil products (ghee, or butter oil)	Vitamin A
Philippines	Filled milk	Vitamins A and D
	Margarine	Vitamins A and D, thiamine
Thailand	Sweetened condensed milk	Vitamin A
Turkey	Table margarine	Vitamins A and D

Source: Darnton-Hill and Nalubola 2002

Fortification has tended to cost less per child than capsule supplementation, though this is based on a limited number of studies, with sugar fortification in Guatemala (see Box 2-4) as the clearest example (Caulfield, Richard et al. 2006). In 1994, fortification of sugar cost an estimated Rs. 7 (US$0.17) per child, and the cost of saving a DALY ranged from Rs. 1,326 to 1,407 (US$33 to US$35), not including such nonfatal effects as improved eye and general health.

In an analysis to determine whether the Philippines should institute a wheat fortification program to complement or replace the long-standing National Vitamin A Supplementation Program described earlier in this chapter, the estimated ongoing costs of wheat fortification included incremental production costs, promotion of the program, internal processing costs, and external monitoring (Fiedler, Dado et al. 2000). In total, it was estimated that fortifying hard wheat flour (the type of flour usually baked in breads) with 490 RAEs per 100 grams would add less than 1 percent to the total cost of milled flour. However, although fortification of the flour with 490 retinol equivalents per 100 grams would be twice as efficient as the supplementation program, the analysis showed that it would still leave 29 percent of children with VAD. Although favoring fortification over supplementation based on a cost analysis, the authors acknowledged that continued supplementation was needed to reach the significant percentage of particularly vulnerable children.

Box 2-4
Fortification Case Study: Sugar in Central America

In the 1970s, Guatemala, Honduras, and Costa Rica launched an effort to fortify sugar with vitamin A. Sugar was chosen as the vehicle because of its low cost, ease of implementation, wide consumption, and the fact that it is centrally produced and then purchased by consumers, rather than grown and processed at home (like corn and other crops). Moreover, the vitamin A in fortified sugar was bioavailable, did not alter the taste, look, or feel (i.e., it was "organoleptically acceptable"), and was stable under Central America's hot, humid conditions and after cooking (Sommer and West 1996).

The Institute of Nutrition of Central America and Panama developed the technology and first introduced fortified sugar in Guatemala in 1975. Initial results were dramatic: vitamin A intake almost tripled and VAD decreased from 22 to 5 percent over a one-year period. Because of this, Guatemala made fortification of sugar mandatory. The effort was halted in 1979 because of civil unrest, lack of enforcement, cost to the industry, and a worldwide sugar glut that undercut the Guatemalan price, but was restarted in the late 1980s.

Costa Rica and Honduras have implemented mandatory sugar fortification at various times since then, and El Salvador has used it since 1994. The technology has been modernized over the years as sugar production has become more automated. A quality-assurance system was developed in Honduras and transferred to the other countries in the 1990s.

Total cost of the program in the late 1990s was Rs. 378 (US$9.40) per metric ton (MT), almost all assumed by the industry and passed on to consumers. In 1998–1999, 7,00,000 MTs of sugar was fortified in El Salvador, Guatemala, and Honduras, serving 2.4 crore (24 million) people. Total cost was Rs. 26 crore (US$6.58 million), broken down as follows: Rs. 12 (US$0.30) per person covered, Rs. 21 (US$0.51) per high-risk person covered, and Rs. 31 (US$0.76) per vulnerable high-risk person covered.

Fortified sugar now provides between 45 and 180 percent of vitamin A reference daily intake to people older than age 3, and about 30 percent to children under age 3 (Dary and Mora 2002).

Some of the lessons learned in this project apply to fortification efforts elsewhere. For example, a review of the project stressed the need for participation of producers from the planning stage, as well as presence of an institution to bring all stakeholders together, adequate legal or statutory instruments, and media campaigns to inform consumers about the benefits of fortification and about identifying and using the fortified foodstuff.

Sources: Mora, Dary et al. 2000; Dary and Mora 2002

Fortification in India

Less than 1 percent of food in India is fortified, although the government, through various ministries and NGOs, has been trying to increase the amount as another way to boost consumption of vitamin A, iron, and other nutrients (Micronutrient Initiative 2005). Some of these efforts are summarized below.

As with supplementation, India was a pioneer in food fortification. In 1962, vitamin A fortification of ghee was made mandatory (Gupta 2000), but the requirement has not been strictly enforced (ACC/SCN 2001). Fortification of vanaspati, a hydrogenated vegetable oil that substitutes for ghee, is also required based on laws from the 1950s (Sridhar 1997), again not universally enforced. Even if vanaspati fortification were more complete, consumption patterns indicate that it would meet the needs of consumers only in the urban north, and although the contribution to daily intake would be significant there, it would not reach the poor (Sridhar 1997). Sommer and West (1996) reported that India developed the technology to fortify tea with vitamin A but with little follow-through in the commercial sector. They note that although fortified tea would not benefit most children, it might raise vitamin A levels of fertile and pregnant women and mothers. Ultra Rice™, a fortified mixture that can be combined and cooked with regular, white rice, has been introduced in India but remains at the testing and pilot stage (Lee, Hamer et al. 2000). This method is practical only where rice is processed centrally, rather than where it is grown and processed on small farms.

The Micronutrient Initiative has supported fortification pilot projects in various states. These projects have included the distribution of fortified flour, oil, salt, and condiments through the Mid-Day Meal Programme to children in parts of Gujarat, Andhra Pradesh, Bihar, and West Bengal; fortified wheat through the Targeted Public Distribution System (TPDS) to low-income households; "nutri-candies" (lozenges fortified with vitamin A, iron, and other nutrients) through Anganwadi centers to children and pregnant and lactating women; a fortified powder called Vita Shakti that is added to rice and lentils; and a powder called Anuka for weaned infants (Micronutrient Initiative 2005). Per capita costs have ranged from Rs. 1.50 (US$.04) for fortified wheat flour to Rs. 55 (US$1.36) for the candies. The Micronutrient Initiative also works with the ICDS in implementing a micronutrient society model on the state level—a legally autonomous entity that is subject to some government oversight but independent of government control (Lakshman 2006). The hope is that these societies have the flexibility of an NGO while maintaining credibility.

The United Nations World Food Programme supported the development of a food blend called IndiaMix, a mixture of wheat and soy fortified with vitamin A and other micronutrients. It has distributed IndiaMix through the ICDS Supplementary Nutrition Programme, principally in Rajasthan but also in other states. A 100-gram serving provides about 80 percent of a child's RDA for vitamin A and iron. In 2000, IndiaMix cost about Rs. 10,859 (US$270) per ton to produce (World Food Programme 2000).

In 1997, the National Federation of Cooperative Sugar Factories, Ltd., partnered with the Micronutrient Initiative on a pilot project to fortify sugar with 12 or 15 mg of vitamin A per kilogram (Marathe 2001). Estimated cost was Rs. 51 (US$1.26) per 100 kg at 15 mg/kg, and Rs. 46 (US$1.15) at 12 mg/kg; the vitamin A was imported, and the cost might have been lower if produced domestically. After the successful completion of the pilot, the sugar factories federation urged the government to grant a tax exemption to fortified sugar to lower its price, noting that the fortified sugar has a yellowish tinge that, combined with a higher price, would make it less attractive to consumers (Damodaran 2002). As of this writing, this exemption had not been granted.

India has also tried other initiatives. One, in the 1960s, was the production and sale of Indian Multi-Purpose Food, a blend of 75 percent edible peanut flour and 25 percent Bengal gram (*Cicer arietinum*, garbanzo bean or chickpea). This food item provided protein and several nutrients, including 3,000 IUs of vitamin A. However, despite a large volume of sales, lack of government support along with poor marketing led to the demise of the program (Achaya 1984). Around the same time, a similar project to fortify dough with tapioca flour also foundered for nontechnical reasons (Achaya 1984). Salt has been a contentious vehicle for supporting iodine fortification in India. A law making it illegal to sell noniodized salt was rescinded after a few years because of arguments relating to personal rights to noniodized salt (Darnton-Hill and Nalubola 2002). The ban has been recently reintroduced, but the ordeal underlies the importance of educating consumers and making sure that the political will is there to follow through.

The Nutrition Syndicate, a leading advocate for food fortification in India, notes that consumer demand is critical if food fortification is to expand in India. The lack of demand may stem from conflicting reports about fortified products. There is also debate in India over the extent of the VAD problem, the efficacy of supplementation, and the safety of fortification, as shown in the case of iodized salt. Regulation of a fairly fragmented market is difficult, and few products are truly universally consumed or centrally produced. In addition, India faces special challenges because of its size: programs that work in one state may not work in states with a different culture and regional foods. Thus, despite the many pilots and other promising studies, vitamin A-fortified foods are not routinely consumed in most of India.

India does have mechanisms that have been used to distribute fortified foods, including the Public Distribution System (PDS) and the TPDS, which subsidize the distribution of wheat, rice, edible oil, kerosene, and sugar through shops in rural and urban areas (Kochar 2005) and could deliver affordable fortified foods to the poor (see Box 2-5). In addition, as noted above, ICDS is designed to provide integrated health, education, and nutrition services; thus, it has been used as a conduit for fortification as well as supplementation. The Mid-Day Meal Programme provides nutritious meals to school-aged children to improve both nutrition and school attendance (Ventatesh Mannar and Sankar 2004).

Box 2-5
The Public Distribution System

The PDS is India's largest antipoverty program, accounting for around 36 percent of the total expenditure on antipoverty and social service programs and 5.2 percent of total government expenditures. PDS evolved in the 1950s and 1960s as a means to stabilize prices of commodities, which were in short supply. With the advent of the Green Revolution and surplus agricultural output, the mission of PDS changed to ensuring access at affordable prices for everyone. The program reaches more than 1 crore (10 million) families and distributes commodities worth more than Rs. 30,000 crore (US$7.5 billion). It cost the government around 21,000 crore ($US5.2 billion) in 2002–2003.

In 1997, the universal approach of PDS was dropped in favor of a more targeted distribution, following budget difficulties and evidence that the program was only marginally useful in increasing welfare and nutrition of poor households. The new TPDS categorizes households as above or below the poverty line and bases distributions on these categories. Although the rules of the program have fluctuated somewhat, the end result is that households below the poverty line are supposed to pay far less for goods than households above the line.

A detailed analysis of the program found that PDS and TPDS had a fairly small effect on the estimated elasticity of caloric intake. The subsidies did little to increase the amount of food eaten, which argues that a large universal system is inefficient and likely to be unsustainable. The study also found that although TPDS targets the poor more effectively than PDS, the amount the poor get is actually less, perhaps because of poor governmental control over the distribution of food, leakage in the system, or problems in distribution. Under TPDS, the only way to get the food is to go to a "fair price shop," which may be far away, and then wait, often for several hours. Thus, even though targeted distribution may have greater potential to reach needy people, realizing this potential is difficult.

Source: Kochar 2005

Food-Based Approaches

As the third strategy to increase vitamin A intake, people can be educated and encouraged to consume more vitamin A-rich foods. These programs may involve increasing the amounts of these foods already consumed as part of normal dietary patterns, or diversifying the diet to include new plant or animal foods that provide the vitamin.

For example, some countries have implemented programs to encourage growing beta-carotene-rich foods for family consumption, or raising small animals or fish stocks (ACC/SCN 2001). Increasing economic prosperity through gardening or other activities can have the secondary benefit of raising incomes so that households can buy a wider variety of nutritious food (Caulfield, Richard et al. 2006). Other projects have focused on home food-processing techniques that retain more vitamin A and on making these often-seasonal foods available throughout more of the year (Ruel and Levin 2000). Nutrition education and social marketing are also recognized as an important component of food-based interventions to maximize results.

Such approaches are particularly promising for those who consume little or no foods that may be fortified because they lack income or access to commercially processed foods. However, relying on diet alone to bolster vitamin A intake is complicated by the inherent differences in the bioavailability of vitamin A, as discussed in Chapter 1, which corresponds to the amount of dietary intake.

Food-Based Approaches Worldwide

As noted in Chapter 1, there is some question about the feasibility of getting enough vitamin A through diet alone, especially for those without access to fortified foods or animal products. Beyond limited bioavailability, dietary strategies that center on home gardens face such vulnerabilities as the environmental and seasonal risks of gardening, the possibility that poor households may instead use the gardens for income-producing crops, and the fact that varied local conditions hamper the creation of national policies or programs to support these activities (Underwood 2000). A further impediment to more widespread funding of community-based food-centered programs is that they are difficult to evaluate: many variables may confound clear findings (Underwood 2004). Despite the need for food-based programs, their effects have not been clearly demonstrated for several possible reasons, including small budgets allocated to evaluation; an assumption that food production or consumption alone, rather than improved nutritional status, is sufficient to show success; and small study populations that make showing the effect on nutritional deficiencies or morbidity difficult to prove (de Pee, Bloem et al. 2000).

Nevertheless, some evidence shows that food-based programs can improve vitamin A status (ACC/SCN 2001). Interventions that promote increased intake of micronutrient-rich foods through social marketing and communications have shown more positive results than earlier home-gardening interventions that did not include an education or communications component (Ruel and Levin 2000). Communications-related components have included radio spots and a social marketing campaign in Indonesia, community-based activities in Thailand, and an education and meals project based in Lima's community kitchens. In Kenya, when two women's groups were introduced to new varieties of sweet potatoes to plant, the group that received nutrition education, lessons on food processing, and technical assistance consumed more vitamin A-rich foods than the group that received minimal support. In fact, a decrease in vitamin A consumption occurred among the latter group (Hagenimana, Anyango Oynga et al. 1999). In Bangladesh, Helen Keller International developed a home gardening project that has shown nutritional as well as economic impacts (Box 2-6).

Research shows that to increase the chances that dietary diversification will improve vitamin A status, several elements must be in place: (1) because carotenoid content varies so widely, based on the species and processing and preparation methods, it is crucial to choose foods with high carotenoid contents that are eaten regularly and prepared in ways to make the carotenoids most bioavailable; (2) seasonal availability and deterioration of beta-carotene during storage must be considered; (3) new foods and food preparations must be acceptable and effective; and (4) nutritional education, communication, and accessibility are crucial (IVACG 2004). These elements may also relate to a consideration of how to successfully introduce biofortified mustard.

Box 2-6
Case Study: Home Food Production in Bangladesh

Efforts over 20 years in Bangladesh lowered the incidence of clinical VAD in children significantly, from 3.5 percent in 1982–1983 to 0.62 percent in 1997–1998 (Helen Keller International 1999). Although supplementation is the main reason for the decline, homestead gardening was also associated with these results.

Helen Keller International, which has focused on VAD in the context of eliminating preventable causes of blindness, first undertook a pilot project in northwest Bangladesh in 1988 that combined the promotion of home gardens with nutrition education. The pilot identified some constraints to participation, such as the need for a reliable supply of seeds and other inputs. In 1993, the program, which expanded to work with the government and NGOs around the country, was designed to overcome the constraints identified in the pilot. In addition to such technical elements as access to seeds, water, and pest control, elements of success included access to capital and credit, technical assistance, and nutrition education and social marketing to change feeding and eating behaviors so that more nutritious crops are grown and eaten.

Helen Keller International also set up a pilot project that included an animal husbandry component along with the vegetable gardening. Model farms were established with household egg production, de-worming tablets for cows to increase their milk production, and fish cultivars and improved fish feed for aquaculture. An evaluation showed that households participating in the program increased their consumption of eggs, fish, and liver significantly, and income from the sale of poultry products was used for other foods and household needs.

Sources: Helen Keller International 1999; Talukder, Kiess et al. 2000

Food-Based Approaches in India

The National Consultation on the Benefits and Safety of Vitamin A Administration that advised against some uses of supplementation (see earlier discussion) expressed strong support for food-based approaches, stating, "production and consumption of vitamin A rich foods must be strongly promoted in the community, particularly among pregnant and lactating women and children" (National Consultation 2001). This promotion has been attempted through many public and private channels. For example, the National Institute of Nutrition provides information on how to augment vitamin A and other micronutrient intake with locally available foods (http://www.ninindia.org/popular.htm).

Some promising projects have targeted vulnerable populations in India. A home gardening project to combat VAD was carried out in Andhra Pradesh (Vijayaraghavan, Nayak et al. 1997). In each study village, one person was trained to serve as a central point to distribute seeds and seedlings, demonstrate correct planting methods, and carry out education programs about the role of home gardening in nutrition. At the district level, a postgraduate trained in nutrition or social sciences monitored and supervised the program. By the end of three years, 65 percent of the households were growing carotene-rich foods in home gardens, compared with 10 percent at the beginning. Unfortunately, despite strong participation and corresponding increases in the consumption of carotene-rich foods, the prevalence of Bitot's spots did not significantly decline, nor were mean serum retinol levels significantly affected. The authors suggest that more fat in the diet or a longer research period may have been needed to see results. They also recommended a "multisectoral strategy" that included supplementation as well as long-term sustainable home gardening.

During the 1980s, the Regional Research Laboratories in Trivandrum was involved in a multicountry effort to maintain the beta-carotene content of red palm oil through the production cycle, an effort that began as far back as the 1930s (Rao 2000). Surveys showed that foods prepared with red palm oil only were moderately accepted but were well accepted when combined with other oils. In a 10-month trial in rural Tamil Nadu, about 400 preschool children ate a noonday meal that incorporated red palm oil.

The snack was acceptable to the children and resulted in a lower prevalence of Bitot's spots by the end of the trial (Sivan 2001).

Why Not India?

India has expressed its commitment to improving its population's nutritional status. The Tenth Five-Year Plan, which covers 2002–2007, calls for increased spending and stepped-up efforts to improve nutrition and reduce health disparities and poverty. This plan follows from many decades of well-intentioned policies and political support to fight malnutrition since Independence, perhaps most famously during the Green Revolution in the late 1960s and 1970s. The National Nutrition Policy in 1993 explicitly linked nutrition with development and mandated that deficiencies of vitamin A, iron, folic acid, and iodine be controlled through "intensified programmes (Government of India 1993)."

Despite the good intentions and strong economic growth, in 2005, the World Bank categorized India, along with 27 other countries, as having achieved "some improvement, but ... not on track" to meet the Millennium Development Goal of eradicating extreme poverty and hunger (World Bank 2005). Why have the interventions described in this chapter— supplementation, fortification, and food-based approaches— had only limited success in reducing VAD, particularly subclinical VAD, in India?

As discussed in Chapter 1, the obvious explanations include the size of the country, the total number of those living in poverty, and gender and caste disparities. Another factor might be the low consumption of meat and dairy products (ACC/SCN 2001). According to U.S. Department of Agriculture (USDA) figures, the per capita consumption of meat products (beef, pork, poultry, and mutton) in developing countries is only about one-third that of industrialized countries (24 kg per capita annually versus 72 kg). India's per capita figure, 2 kg annually, is just a small fraction of even developing countries' already-low average. According to a 1991 survey by the National Sample Survey Organisation, daily meat consumption in India ranged from 1 g per capita among the lowest-income class to about 14 g among the highest. Milk consumption ranged from less than 10 g among the lowest-income class to more than 400 g among the highest

(Hopper 1999). As a point of comparison, the Indian Council of Medical Research recommends a daily consumption of 280 g per day—an amount that the poor do not even begin to achieve.

Other factors are suggested by results of the 2003 NNMB survey. When the bureau looked at why supplementation coverage was low in the eight states it surveyed, slightly more than half of the adults surveyed said that supplementation was not offered, and about one-third said they were not aware of the program. Very few cited such reasons as inconvenience or refusal (NNMB 2003b). Income also does not completely explain the situation, since some states with relatively high rates of poverty, such as Bihar and Jharkhand, are among those with higher supplementation coverage. Some observers look at on-the-ground implementation, noting that strong local government and civil society support make the difference (Micronutrient Initiative 2005).

The NNMB survey also indicated a low level of knowledge about the role of diet in preventing VAD. Overall, fewer than one-half of the mothers questioned in the eight states surveyed were aware of night blindness. Fewer than one-quarter knew that dietary changes could prevent VAD, and even fewer were aware of the types of foods that could be used. Only 13.2 percent reported that they had received nutrition education on VAD. Given that nutrition education has been found to be an integral part of food-based strategies to reduce VAD, India will need to find new ways to communicate this important information to households, particularly to women, if diets are to be meaningfully altered to include more vitamin A-rich foods.

In a review of the status of vitamin A supplementation and other micronutrient programs, a senior official of the National Institute of Nutrition posited reasons behind the difficulties in achieving success in India. He identified seven "constraints and obstacles": (1) inadequate supplies; (2) poor outreach; (3) irregular distribution; (4) lack of orientation for administrators; (5) absence of community participation; (6) absence of nutrition education; and (7) nonutilization of resources, in part due to a high illiteracy rate. His suggestions for improving vitamin A intake in India included looking at new delivery systems, social marketing, encouragement of home gardening, and stepped-up nutrition education (Vijayaraghavan 2002).

Despite promising activities in various communities, the PDS, TPDS, and ICDS are not realizing their potential for improving nutritional status. One study indicated that only 22 percent of PDS expenditures reached the poorest populations, and TPDS has not improved on that figure (ACC/SCN 2001). TPDS was designed, as the name suggests, to "target" more food aid to the poor, yet it is used by only a small proportion of those eligible (Kochar 2005). Likewise, a study of the role of ICDS in improving child nutrition in India found gaps between the program's policy intentions and implementation (Gragnolati, Shekar et al. 2005). The principal gaps were the program's focus on the day-to-day provision of food to the detriment of nutrition education and other longer-term activities; relatively less attention to girls, lower castes, and poorer villages, all of whom are at higher risk of undernutrition; and less funding and coverage for the poorest states and those with the highest levels of undernutrition. An evaluation of the Mid-Day Meal Programme in Karnataka showed a positive impact on school attendance but little impact on nutritional status; in any event, the program targets older children than those targeted in most vitamin A programs (Laxmaiah, Sarm et al. 1999).

In designing strategies to improve nutrition, including vitamin A status, some of the broader considerations to bear in mind are suggested by two studies of poor children, one in rural Tamil Nadu (Shekar, Habicht et al. 1991) and the other in urban Mumbai (Merchant and Udipi 1997). In 42 Tamil Nadu villages, more than 3,000 children were monitored over 12 months and classified as "positive deviants" (high end of the growth spectrum), median growers, or "negative deviants" (low end of the growth spectrum). Through follow-up research, the authors found that different factors characterized the households of children with greater or lesser growth. Strong growth among children was associated with 23 variables, including landownership, age of the mother, and the number of hours the mother spent working. Sex of the child (female) and lower maternal wealth were among the traits associated with lower rates of growth.

The Mumbai study applied this growth framework in an urban slum context. According to the study, the ability of the mother to use available resources wisely was the main determinant of whether her child had a positive growth pattern. These mothers were more likely to make such choices as spending available income on nutritious foods or seeking medical help when necessary. The decisionmaking power of the mothers within the household also influenced their children's growth: the children of mothers with more decisionmaking power generally thrived more. The authors pointed to the need for parental education, as well as assistance to mothers to prioritize their problems, effectively use resources, and put knowledge into practice. Although these factors fall outside the scope of the investigation of the feasibility of biofortified mustard, they are worth bearing in mind to achieve the ultimate goal—improved vitamin A status of children and women. The World Bank notes that "a good way to ensure new practices make sense is to see what … poor women with well-nourished children are doing right" (World Bank 2005).

Summary

Supplementation. India was one of the first countries in the world to launch a supplementation program, but its program currently reaches only about one-third of the children who need it. Coverage varies greatly by state. Reasons for the variation and limited coverage rates include a well-publicized case of hypervitaminosis (overdosing of vitamin A) in Assam, combined with a lack of scientific consensus about supplementation campaigns and dispersed populations without access to health facilities.

Fortification. About 1 percent of food in India is fortified with vitamin A, although the government, Micronutrient Initiative, and other organizations have made efforts to fortify products that range from vanaspati and rice to candy for children. A lack of enforcement, resistance by producers to incur additional costs not borne by their competitors, and the dispersed nature of production and processing facilities for many common foods have impeded more widespread fortification efforts.

Food-based approaches. Even though home gardening and dietary diversification efforts have been made in India, continued low levels of consumption of animal products by lower-income households seem to inhibit significant increases in vitamin A intake through increased gardening alone. Other food-based projects, such as including beta-carotene rich red palm oil into noonday meals for children, have been shown to be promising, but have only been attempted at a local level.

Notes

[1] A reduction in child mortality is the ultimate measure of success, but coverage is used as the indicator because it is difficult to distinguish the role of vitamin A in mortality data.

[2] Variations in the costs per death averted by country can be explained in part by the campaign strategy used (one or two doses in a single year) and by the number and proportion of the child population targeted and reached. Variations in child mortality rates between countries also accounted for some of the variations; incremental costs per death averted declined exponentially as child mortality rates increased.

[3] In the United States, adoption of fortified salt and milk and enriched bread faced similar obstacles (Bishai and Nalubola 2002).

CHAPTER 3

Mustard and Its Potential to Improve Health in India

Mustard plants (genus *Brassica*, which also includes broccoli, cabbage, cauliflower, radishes, arugula, and turnips) are believed to have been first cultivated in the foothills of the Himalayan Mountains more than 5,000 years ago, and thus mustard is one of the oldest crops in human civilization. Mustard plants are erect, leafy, flowering plants that can grow to about 1 to 2 meters and produce bright yellow flowers and seed pods. Consumers, processors, and state statisticians in India consider all brown-seeded mustard the same, but technically, the mustard crop comprises genetically distinct species, including *Brassica campestris, B. juncea*, and *B. nigra*. Of the three major varieties, *B. juncea* is the most prevalent, but Toria, a variety of *B. campestris*, is grown extensively in India's east and in the far north (Pental, Pradhan et al. 2001; Sengupta and Das 2003). The most common variety of *B. juncea* is Varuna, which was released some 30 years ago but has yet to be surpassed in yield by any new variety (Pental, Pradhan et al. 2001). All major varieties can be genetically modified through biotechnology to express higher levels of carotenoids, and beta-carotene specifically (Singh, pers. comm.).

Mustard seed was used by the ancient Chinese and Greeks because of its medicinal properties,[1] but it was likely the Romans who first ground mustard seeds into a paste similar to modern mustard sauce. Mustard seeds can also be used to garnish or spice food directly, as well as pressed into oil. In India, the vast majority of mustard seed is consumed as oil—in cooking or pickling or as seasoning.[2]

To assess the potential of biofortified mustard to improve vitamin A status in India, one must understand how mustard seed moves from the farm to the potential target group—vitamin A-deficient consumers, particularly children and women. In this chapter we trace mustard oil's path in India from the production of mustard seed to oil processing to consumption. We then examine how mustard use corresponds to areas where VAD is a public health concern and examine its potential. Lastly, we examine some of the challenges associated with adopting this technology.

Production

India was the world's fifth-largest producer of major oilseeds[3] in 2005–2006, producing around 3.066 crore (30.66 million) metric tons, or 8 percent of the world total, behind the United States, Brazil, China, and Argentina (USDA 2006a). Mustard-rapeseed (grouped together in most agricultural statistics) accounted for about 22 percent of India's oilseed production in that period (see Figure 3-1).

Figure 3-1. Major Oilseed Production in India, 2005–2006

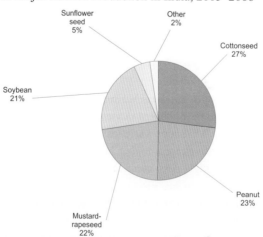

Source: USDA 2006a

Mustard-rapeseed is produced almost entirely domestically, with imports typically accounting for less than 1 percent of production. In 2005–2006, imports accounted for just 17,000 MTs of a total harvest of 6.5 crore (65 million) MTs, an increase of more than 350 percent since 1964 (Figure 3-2). However, the dramatic increase in production has been due more to acreage expansion than to yield improvements, for mustard-rapeseed yield per hectare in India is only about one-half the world average (Dohlman, Persaud et al. 2003). More broadly, yields in all India's major oilseed crops are significantly below world averages. The yields are constrained mainly because most oilseed production depends on monsoon rainfall, which can be erratic. Moreover, farmers face significant price risk, since the government often sets minimum price supports that are too low, does not enforce them, or makes them difficult for farmers to obtain. Because of these considerable risks, farmers, who typically operate at small scales and have limited resources, are hesitant to invest in improved seeds, fertilizer, and pesticides (USDA 2006c). In addition, mustard-rapeseed production has been hurt by high minimum price supports for wheat, which grows under similar conditions and thus can be an attractive economic alternative for farmers.

Figure 3-2. Mustard-Rapeseed Domestic Production, Imports, and Domestic Consumption in India, 1964–2006

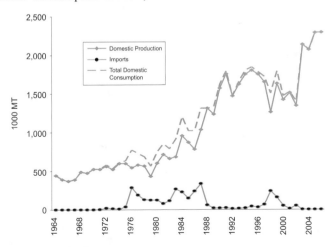

Source: USDA 2006b

Table 3-1. Area, Production, and Yield of Rapeseed and Mustard, 2001–2002, by State

	Area (million ha)	Percentage of total area	Production (MT)	Percentage of total production	Yield (kg/ha)
Rajasthan	1.84	36.29	1.94	38.19	1,056
Uttar Pradesh	0.85	16.77	0.85	16.73	998
Haryana	0.54	10.65	0.80	15.75	1,488
Madhya Pradesh	0.51	10.06	0.46	9.06	908
West Bengal	0.44	8.68	0.34	6.69	766
Assam	0.27	5.33	0.14	2.76	504
Gujarat	0.25	4.93	0.29	5.71	1,182
Bihar	0.09	1.78	0.08	1.57	839
Punjab	0.05	0.99	0.06	1.18	1,200
Others	0.23	4.54	0.12	2.36	—*
All India	5.07	100	5.08	100	1,002

Source: Government of India 2004

* Since area and production are low in these other states, yield rate is not worked out.

Although mustard can grow in various terrains, it thrives best in fertile, well-drained, loamy soils and at cool temperatures of about 8° to 10°C (Oplinger, Oelke et al. 1991). Therefore, mustard is a winter crop, usually planted in October and harvested in March, and mostly in the cooler north, particularly in the states of Rajasthan, Uttar Pradesh, Haryana, West Bengal, Madhya Pradesh, Gujarat, and Assam (see Table 3-1).

Roughly 4 crore to 5 crore (40 million to 50 million) farmers grow mustard in India. Most farms (about 90 percent) are small, growing only about 2 hectares (5 acres) of mustard per year and producing most of their crop for household consumption. The larger farms, about 15 to 20 hectares (40 to 50 acres), use mechanized equipment and sell a portion of their crops (Singh 2006).

The overall cost of growing mustard is approximately Rs. 3,000 per hectare (US$74). The cost can be higher if a farmer uses a nutrient management protocol to guide the application of fertilizers, manure, and other nutrients, but use of these protocols is rare. Mustard farmers buy seeds from nearby local sources as well as from large seed-producing companies. The cost varies from as little as Rs. 30 (US$0.75) per kg, when seeds are bought from an NGO or the government, to as much as Rs. 150–

200 (US$3.72–4.97) per kg from commercial seed companies, including Pioneer, Pro-Agro, and Mahyco, the three largest. Most farmers purchase new seed each year rather than save their own to sow the next growing season because they lack optimal seed storage facilities. Moreover, farmers typically hedge their bets and produce more than one variety each year. These varieties intercross and result in hybrid seeds with fewer of the advantageous characteristics of the parent generation. In any event, growing mustard does not require a lot of seed and, thus, seeds represent a small percentage of total input costs; one hectare of mustard requires about 3 kg of seed. Seeds are typically bought at seed festivals, known as melas, which are also a source of general agricultural information. Melas are held in the larger towns, so farmers from a small village often send a representative to collect information and purchase seeds on their behalf (Yadav, pers. comm.). These purchase patterns could come into play in developing a strategy to reach farmers with biofortified mustard seed.

Seeds mature about 90 to 95 days after planting and yield about 20 quintals (about 2,000 kg) per hectare. As with other crops in India, mustard is produced at all levels of technological sophistication, and containers to protect the crop from sun, heat, rain, and pests range from gunny bags, earthen pots, and bamboo baskets to steel bins. Transportation of the harvest to market also ranges widely; farmers may transport their crop in head loads, on the backs of pack animals, or in carts, trucks, or other mechanized transport.

Farmers generally sell their crop directly after harvesting because of the unavailability or high cost of adequate storage facilities. To even out the resulting cyclical downturns in price, the government has constructed godowns (warehouses) to store crops for a later sale date. In addition, several public entities are involved in purchasing the crop to avoid a price drop, in particular the National Agricultural Cooperative Marketing Federation and oilseed cooperatives under the National Dairy Development Board (Saha, Sinha et al. 2004). It is estimated that a farmer can receive about Rs. 1,700 (US$42) per quintal through a sale to the government at what is called the Market Support Price, and Rs. 1,500–1,600 (US$37–39) on the open market. Thus, farmers could gross approximately Rs. 34,000 (US$845) per acre if they sold to the government. However, many farmers do not sell to the government despite the higher price because the process is time-consuming, taking them away from their farms, and fraught with uncertainty due to bureaucratic malfeasance (Singh 2006).

Processing

Around 90 percent of the mustard seed grown in India is used to make oil. Oil is extracted from seeds by crushing and then pressing them slowly. Unlike other oils in India, mustard is cold-pressed and unrefined; this process retains the isothiocyanates, which give the oil a pungency that consumers value, especially in rural areas (Singh 2006).

Processing Facilities

In ascending order of efficiency and yield, mustard oil is produced in the home using a mortar and pestle; in small village-based mills, known as ghanis, for personal consumption and local sale; in small-scale expeller facilities; and in large factories. Though no reliable estimates exist about the extent of home production, anecdotally, quite a bit is processed in this manner (Singh 2006).

Ghanis are the most numerous processing facility (about 1,50,000), but they accounted for less than 5 percent of total oil output in the 1990s because of their low yield. Crushing time is from 2 to 5 hours, with a yield of oil of only about 30 percent. Ghanis have an average output of 60 kg per day, often operating at just 10 percent capacity. The Technology Mission on Oilseeds, Pulses and Maizes in the Department of Agriculture and Cooperation is implementing a program to modernize processing and replace ghanis with mechanical expellers to get fuller recovery of oil from the seed and reduce labor time. However, one attraction of hand-milled oil for consumers is its pungency, in addition to the low capital costs for the ghani operator.

Small-scale expellers dominate the market in rural India. Farmers who take their harvest to these local facilities generally keep some oil for household consumption as well as oilcake for animal feed, and sell the rest (TERI 2006). Small-scale expellers operate at about 30 percent capacity and can produce about 200 kg per hour, accounting for around 58 percent of all domestic edible oil output but only about 20 percent of mustard oil output. Although more efficient than ghanis, they also lose a significant portion of the crop during processing, especially because few are integrated with solvent extraction, so oil and meal production is lost.

Large manufacturers with solvent extractors operate primarily in Rajasthan, Uttar Pradesh, Haryana, and Punjab. These manufacturers purchase seed from a mundi (seed dealer) at the lowest price (including the mundi fee), often across state lines, even though they must pay additional taxes if they purchase seeds from out of state. The large mills operating in these states account for around 75 percent of mustard oil production (Singh 2006). Many mills operate according to the "cluster" concept, in which there is a localized concentration of mills. In these larger mills, large stone crushers (kolus) enable cold pressing production, which produces oil and a kolu cake. The cakes are then fed through expellers, which use solvents to get the rest of the oil. The first-pressed oil is the purest and most expensive, but most oil on the market is a combination of the two methods.

Even though large manufacturers are more efficient, small-scale expellers and ghanis dominate mustard oil processing. This is largely because of government regulatory and trade policies, including plant scale restrictions, movement and storage restrictions, credit controls, taxes and tax incentives, and restrictions on futures trading (Dohlman, Persaud et al. 2003; USDA 2006c).

Storage Issues

Mustard oil has a shelf life of up to one year but is seldom kept for that long before consumption. Instead, it is distributed quickly along the supply chain from processor to market. The annual pickling season takes place from July to August, during which demand is highest. Mustard oil moves rapidly from processor to market because of the high demand during these two months. Processors typically keep the oil after extraction for a maximum of four to five days because they lack sufficient storage capacity.

The feasibility of biofortified mustard depends in part on the packaging and storage of oil because of potential losses of vitamin A content. Studies have been conducted to measure vitamin A losses when other types of vitamin A-fortified oils are stored (Favaro, Ferreira et al. 1991). If kept in a sealed, dark container, soybean and some other oils keep most of their vitamin A content for about nine months in lab conditions at 20° to 25°C and in transport in the low- to mid-30°C range. These studies did not test under the extreme heat of the Indian summer, nor did they look specifically at mustard oil (TERI 2006).

Because light breaks down vitamin A in fortified oils, mustard oil, if made from biofortified seed, would need to be stored and transported in sealed, dark containers. As discussed more fully below, consumers purchase oil in either branded or "loose" form. Branded oil (e.g., sold in liters or other quantities for households to use over a duration of weeks or months) would have to be bottled and sold in opaque containers; bulk oil, which is typically sold in small quantities over a few days, would need to be stored properly by the vender or other distributor (such as ICDS or other government agency) in large barrels or other light-blocking containers.

Consumption

Mustard-rapeseed oil has long been one of the most consumed edible oils in India and currently is third, after palm and soybean oil (Figure 3-3), even though most mustard is consumed only in the north.

Figure 3-3. Total Domestic Consumption of Edible Oil, 1972–2006, by Type

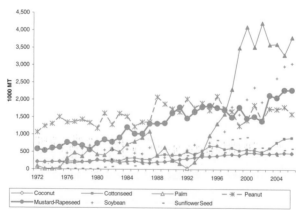

Note: Consumption for 2006 is an estimate.
Source: USDA 2006b

Consumption of mustard oil has grown about 5 percent per year for the past 40 years and currently stands at some 2.3 MTs annually. Across many northern states, average consumption exceeds 30 grams per person per month, but this statistic masks both large differences between states and differences within them. Differences in state averages can vary by as much as one-fold in states that are fairly close to each other, and differences within states occur between rural and urban consumers, as well as between different classes (Figure 3-4). The pattern of consumption across classes suggests that mustard oil is a fairly integral part of many Indian households, regardless of income, though at higher income levels there seems to be a switch to more expensive oils (Dohlman, Persaud et al. 2003).

Although consumption of mustard oil is typically more prevalent in rural areas, total consumption is usually higher in urban areas. In addition, urban households are more likely to use branded oil, and rural households are more likely to consume unbranded (loose) oil (Figure 3-5). This is largely because branded oils cost around Rs. 60–70 per kg, while loose oil costs Rs. 48–50 per kg (IMRB 2006). Despite being called the "poor man's oil," mustard oil is roughly double the cost of other oils, such as palm, ricebran, or soybean. This higher price, combined with its pungency, also makes it fairly easy for producers to adulterate it with other, less costly oils (Singh 2006). The government has made a push toward more packaged oil since 1998, when loose mustard oil was adulterated with argemone, a poisonous additive, causing a number of illnesses (Shiva 2001).

Figure 3-4. Monthly per Capita Purchases of Mustard Oil by Household Income in Rural and Urban Households of Rajasthan, Uttar Pradesh, Bihar, and Madhya Pradesh, 2005

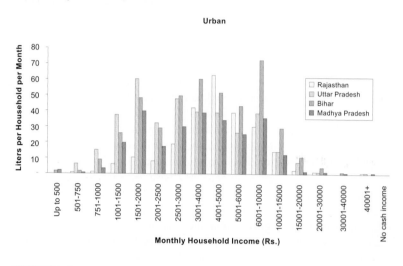

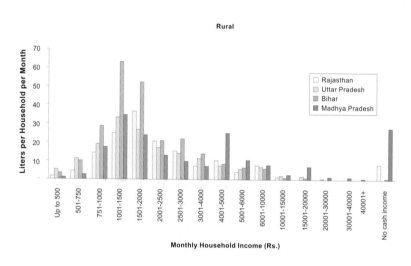

Source: IMRB 2006

Figure 3-5. Percentage of Households that Purchased Mustard Oil in Rural and Urban Areas of Rajasthan, Uttar Pradesh, Bihar, and Madhya Pradesh in 2005

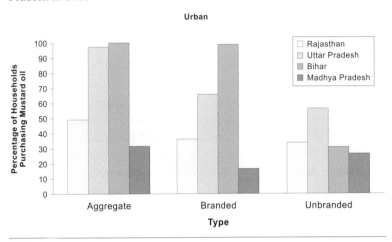

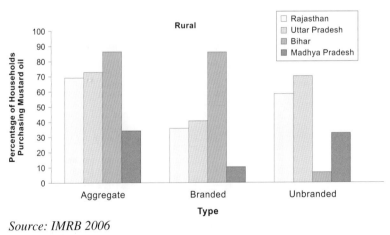

Source: IMRB 2006

Most mustard oil (around 90 percent) is used for cooking, and the rest is used for pickling and consumption as raw oil (sareson-ka-thal, "oil of mustard") directly on foods. According to reports, in rural areas, food is cooked at fairly low heat to maintain the pungency of the oil; in urban areas, pungency is less desirable and food is cooked at higher temperatures

(Singh 2006). This is important because studies on red palm oil, soybean oil, and vanaspati indicate that the primary determinants of how much vitamin A is lost in cooking are the temperature, length of time if fried, and how often the oil is reused (TERI 2006). Duration and temperature of cooking affect vitamin A content, with lower temperatures and one or no reuse resulting in the highest retention.

Fitting the Pieces Together: Vitamin A Deficiency and Mustard Oil Consumption

To justify the expense of introducing biofortified mustard on a commercial scale, there must be an overlap between those who consume mustard oil and the populations most vulnerable to VAD. Thus, a close examination of the intersection of the prevalence of VAD with mustard production and consumption is necessary. In this section, we explore the extent of this overlap, the state of the production of biofortified mustard, and potential measures to extend the reach of biofortified mustard.

Mustard Use and Vitamin A Deficiency

Mustard oil is consumed in every state where a VAD problem is indicated by the presence of Bitot's spots (Figure 3-6).

Figure 3-6. Mustard Oil Consumption and Prevalence of Bitot's Spots, by State

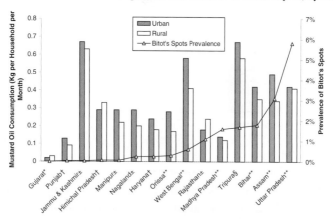

Sources: Consumption data: NSS 2001; Bitot's Spots Prevalence: *NNMB 2002; **NNMB 2003a; ±Toteja, Singh et al. 2001; †NIN 2001; §Chakravarty and Ghosh 2000

Because VAD is primarily a disease of the poor, it is important to further examine the breakdown of mustard consumption and production within these states. Especially in rural areas, mustard oil consumption among the poor is closely tied to household production. Even households with no cash income consume at least small amounts of mustard oil, which suggests the need to tie production and consumption and to get biofortified seed to home growers and local producers.

On the other hand, some states with high prevalence levels of Bitot's spots consume large amounts of mustard oil brought in from mustard-producing states. This suggests that production at regional and national levels is important, too, since people in many states obtain their mustard oil from other places. In other words, both large commercial growers and small producers may need to grow biofortified mustard if the oil is to reach the poor in different situations.

Status of Biofortification

Genetic recombinant technology can be used to induce or enhance the expression of provitamin A carotenoids in plant foods. Like chemically fortified foods, GM biofortified products could potentially provide sustained sources of vitamin A. The GM product that is furthest along in its research and development is vitamin A-enhanced rice, so-called golden rice, but its potential to reduce VAD has yet to be established. In fact, its effectiveness may be limited by its yellowish appearance and the targeted population's low fat intake and consequent insufficient biological absorption of carotenoids (Dawe, Robertson et al. 2002; Egana 2003; Zimmerman and Qaim 2004).

In India, The Energy and Resources Institute, with technical support from the Monsanto Company and Michigan State University, has reported the development of transgenic lines of Indian mustard (*Brassica juncea*) with enhanced levels of beta-carotene expressed in the seed mesocarp (Shewmaker, Sheehy et al. 1999; Agricultural Biotechnology Support Project 2003). When processed into mustard oil, the fat-soluble carotenoids in the mesocarp are retained in the oil (Shewmaker, Sheehy et al. 1999). Biofortified mustard oil has the potential to alleviate VAD in India not only because of its high content of bioavailable provitamin A, but also because mustard oil is commonly used and consumed by the economically disadvantaged members of Indian society, who are more susceptible to VAD, in both urban and rural areas of states where VAD is prevalent.

The mustard research builds on Monsanto-supported research that achieved a 50-fold increase in carotenoids in the mature seed of canola (*Brassica napus*) (Shewmaker, Sheehy et al. 1999). The research done to date, however, shows that although transformations were successful in perhaps 7 or 8 plants per 100 in the case of canola, only about 1 per 100 mustard plants were successfully transformed, thus adding to the costs. In addition, GM canola and mustard seeds both produce slightly lower yields than their conventional counterparts, in the range of about 10 percent under ideal growing conditions (George, pers. comm). Other current research into GM mustard seed has focused on improving productivity. The Centre for Genetic Manipulation of Crop Plants and Department of Genetics at the University of Delhi South Campus developed two hybrids in mustard DMH-1 and DMH-11, which have, on average, 30 percent more productivity over the current best national varieties.

Although outside the scope of this analysis, the political and legal environment for GM products must be taken into account. The government has generally been supportive of biotechnology, with political leaders publicly praising its potential to address nutritional deficiencies. The Genetic Engineering Approval Committee, under the Ministry of Environment and Forests, is supposed to coordinate research in India. Yet at the same time, regulations have been put into place that can restrict research. A 2006 Supreme Court decision allowed for field trials of GM mustard to continue at the University of Delhi, despite regulations to restrain new approvals of GM crops (Reuters 2006).

Box 3-1
Introduction of Biofortified Mustard Seed

Both public and private institutions support producers and processors and might be avenues to introduce biofortified mustard seed.

- The Mustard Research and Promotion Council has operated since 1998 and has a government-approved laboratory for testing mustard oil. It runs a small pilot project to encourage the production of organic mustard oil and operates trial fields to experiment with different varieties of mustard. It reportedly has high credibility among farmers (Singh 2006).

● The State Oilseeds Growers Federation Ltd., District Oilseeds Growers Cooperatives, and Village Oilseed Growers Society all operate to promote production.

● The National Research Centre for Rapeseed-Mustard, in Bharatpur, Rajasthan, is affiliated with the Indian Council of Agricultural Research.

● The government can disseminate information about production and processing through its Market Research and Information Network in the Directorate of Marketing and Inspection.

● In addition, to reach vitamin A-deficient populations in areas where mustard oil is not normally consumed, especially the south, biofortified mustard oil could be blended with other oils, such as groundnut oil (TERI 2006).

Sources: Singh 2006, TERI 2006

Biofortification Potential

Before investigating whether biofortified mustard seed is worth the economic investment, we examine whether it can improve the vitamin A status of currently deficient populations. The answer depends on the different delivery mechanisms to children and pregnant and lactating women, and the extent of their consumption.

How much mustard oil would be needed to achieve 100 percent RDA of vitamin A? A conservative estimate suggests that the beta-carotene content of biofortified mustard would be around 185 µg/g (TERI 2006); more generous estimates suggest that the amount could be at least 600 µg/ g (May 1994; Shewmaker, Sheehy et al. 1999).[4] Since beta-carotene has a retinol equivalency ratio of 2:1 in oil (Zimmerman and Qaim 2004), the effective concentration of vitamin A would be between 92.5 µg and 300 µg per gram of oil. Assuming that all cooking oil is biofortified mustard oil and that high temperatures do not reduce the amount of beta-carotene (both favorable assumptions), a child would need approximately 1 to 4 grams of oil per day (about a teaspoon) to meet the full RDA requirement of 400 µg/ day, with no other sources of vitamin A. However, most children consume at least some amount of vitamin A from other sources, which suggests that even if the concentration of beta-carotene in the oil is less, small dosage levels could still increase their intake to recommended daily values. Thus biofortification, if implemented on a large scale, could significantly improve the vitamin A status of currently deficient populations.

Technology Adoption

Although biofortification may be able to significantly improve the vitamin A status of a population, it faces some inherent challenges. An important advantage of biofortification is that like traditional fortification, it does not rely on bureaucratic or operational efficiency to reach underserved populations, but instead relies on market forces to reach consumers of mustard oil. However, this advantage is balanced against some significant implementation challenges: mustard farmers must be willing to adopt biofortified mustard varieties, and vitamin A-deficient consumers must be willing to consume sufficient quantities of a product that may look different from nonfortified mustard.

The challenges of technology adoption by farmers and consumers are not novel to biofortification, and we can draw some useful lessons from the past. Traditional fortification efforts in the United States succeeded for three important reasons.[5] First, there was a high degree of market concentration among food producers that both helped lower the cost of fortification through scale economies and increased the reliability of monitoring and compliance. Second, fortification was achieved without significant legislative involvement: it was based on public-private partnerships that worked without formal regulation. For example, there is no federal or state government regulation requiring milk to be fortified with vitamin D, but this is the norm throughout the United States. In fact, the experience with iodine fortification of salt in India is a good example of how well-intentioned legislative efforts can fail if regulatory capacity is weak and producers see no benefit. Third, fortification succeeded because of a cultural shift in which consumers perceived the benefit of fortified food and demanded it. Consumer awareness of the health risks associated with micronutrient deficiencies and demand for fortification was created through media campaigns and community mobilization.

In an environment with many small-scale producers[6], fortification is a challenge to implement. Biofortification gets around this challenge by embedding the technology in the raw material—mustard seed. The second and third aspects of the U.S. experience reflect the need for both a "push" strategy to increase the attractiveness of fortification to growers and producers and a "pull" strategy to increase the demand for the fortified oil. Here we discuss how these experiences translate to the Indian context for biofortification.

Technology Adoption by Mustard Growers

A push strategy must rely not only on greater adoption of biofortified mustard by farmers, but also on efforts by mustard oil producers to buy biofortified seed and package biofortified mustard oil as a nutritionally enhanced product.

Indian farmers have been willing to adopt new technologies, such as high-yielding varieties of wheat and rice during the Green Revolution and Bt cotton (with a gene for *Bacillus thuringiensis*, a natural pesticide) in more recent years, when they recognize the benefits of technology adoption. Munshi (2004) found that farmers were slower to adopt high-yielding varieties when growing conditions were relatively heterogeneous (such as for rice). Social information was likely to be more useful when there were contiguous growing areas with relatively homogeneous growing conditions as is the case for mustard.[7] In addition, District Agricultural Offices and organizations like the Mustard Research and Promotion Council can play a role in the adoption process (see Box 3-1).

Promotion efforts are necessary, but farmers may still not be willing to adopt the new technology unless they receive yield benefits or a higher price (or alternatively, a lower price of inputs). There are two ways forward: a higher level of engagement in which a biofortification agency subsidizes producers through a combination of purchase price and/or inputs, or a lower level of engagement that subsidizes seed production alone. Both require a certain degree of involvement and funding by the government or a bilateral or multilateral donor. In either approach, subsidizing purchases of biofortified mustard for target populations by distributing the products to them for free or at reduced prices requires the same level of program involvement as supplementation and fails to capitalize on market forces. Therefore, there is little advantage to a biofortification strategy (whether or not intensive) that has to intervene to ensure the last-mile connectivity with the target consumer.

Vertically Integrated Biofortified Mustard Production and Distribution

Under a higher level of engagement, a formal biofortification agency would directly subsidize growing of biofortified mustard through a combination of purchase price and/or subsidized inputs. A higher support price for biofortified mustard output is one solution, with a subsidized entity buying these seeds at a higher price. The agency (or a commissioned private company) would then be responsible for converting the purchased seed into packaged oil and distributing it through private sector channels at a subsidized price competitive with or below that of regular mustard oil. A useful model for such vertical integration in India is the tobacco industry, which frequently directly engages with tobacco farmers both to lower cost and to improve the quality of tobacco cultivation. A vertically integrated program could also target the biofortified mustard oil to vitamin A-deficient populations through specific programs, but it is likely that a program of traditional fortification could do this just as well: there are no particular benefits of biofortification using this model.

A vertically integrated plan would require significant financial resources and has potential drawbacks. For one, subsidy programs can easily come to be seen as the entitlement of whatever constituency receives them. Even if the subsidy is supposed to be phased out, it may become entrenched. Another consideration is that people affected by micronutrient deficiencies may be both consumers and producers of local agricultural products. If nutritionally enhanced foods are imported into agricultural regions, local people may benefit as consumers but suffer as producers from the increased competition from foreign products.

A Market-Based Approach

A lower level of engagement could be achieved by subsidizing seed production alone while leaving oil production and distribution to the market. Such a program could offer free seeds (versus the current practice, in which most farmers buy their seeds from seed companies during melas). The program could also target the seed subsidies to areas that both grow and consume large quantities of mustard and also have high concentrations of target populations. This program could engage more strongly on the "pull" side through advertising and community mobilization in areas of high VAD prevalence.

The market-based approach would require substantially less financial and organizational investment than the vertical program. It would have the benefit of mixing biofortified mustard with the rest of the mustard oil supply. There are a few challenges, however. First, a significantly high number of mustard growers must adopt the seeds. Without this, the effect of vitamin A biofortification will be diluted by nonbiofortified mustard and will not significantly alter vitamin A intake in affected populations. Second, growers may be reluctant to plant biofortified seed if there is no ready buyer for the harvest and if oil producers consider the seeds inferior to traditional seeds. Third, a significant proportion of the benefits of vitamin A enrichment may accrue to nontarget households that already get vitamin A from other sources, though as the cost-effectiveness analysis in Chapter 4 shows, the program is likely to be beneficial even if it implicitly subsidizes nontarget populations.

Technology Acceptance by Consumers

The type and duration of information provision required to generate consumer acceptance will vary according to the physiological effects a product induces. Medicines for the treatment of acute conditions may be "experience goods"; once a customer has tried them and discovered that they work, she will purchase them again when required. On the other hand, a customer may have to take on faith the assertion that consuming biofortified mustard will forestall chronic conditions. The time span over which effects occur, as well as the number of confounding factors, may preclude individual customers from identifying the benefits of the GM product.

It is important in planning a policy to provide information to customers so that they understand the health and economic benefits they stand to realize. This would require investing in a campaign to educate the public about the importance of micronutrients and consumption of fortified mustard. Rich experience from other public health campaigns in India can inform the effort.

It may also be important to consider what devices will make pronouncements credible. The substantial economic literature on advertising emphasizes that talk alone is cheap. A credible assertion is secured by some "reputational capital"—that is, by the imprimatur of a person or organization with something to lose by being proved wrong. In the U.S. fortification experience, the military and state medical associations played this role. Medical associations in India could take the lead, but it is not clear how much experience they have in taking on public health challenges. Another alternative is for NGOs like the Rotary or Lion's Clubs to promote the benefits of dietary micronutrients.

Issues of credibility can be complex when the improved product is not easily distinguished, but vitamin A-biofortified oil is darker than the traditional product. Food adulteration is not unknown in India, and it is possible that mustard oil could be artificially colored to fake biofortification. If the nutritional attributes of a particular product are not obvious on inspection, consumers must be offered some reliable seal or insignia to identify the enhanced product. The problems of implementing such a scheme are further exacerbated in regions where illiteracy is high and manufacturers routinely counterfeit their products.

Thus, significant hurdles to technology adoption by growers and acceptance by consumers must be overcome to ensure that the projected gains of vitamin A biofortification are attained. These challenges are no less daunting than those facing traditional fortification or supplementation, but they are different. They point to the need to adopt a multiplicity of approaches to the VAD problem in India.

Summary

Mustard production. In many northern states, mustard is grown on small farms and farmers buy their seeds at government-sponsored festivals, and large fractions of seed are planted for home and local use. Most mustard varieties are considered capable of being biofortified, which suggests that it may be fairly easy to introduce large amounts of biofortified seed into the market with little disruption.

Processing. Because of government regulations and market structure, most mustard oil processing takes place in small, local facilities. Traditional fortification would therefore be difficult to achieve on a large scale, since the government has little power to enforce regulations or money to train the many operators. Biofortification allows the seed itself to contain the vitamin A, so even home-based processing—which is thought to be extensive—would produce mustard oil high in vitamin A.

Consumption. Consumption of mustard oil overlaps in many areas where VAD is a public health concern. Preliminary estimates suggest that only small amounts of mustard oil are necessary to significantly raise vitamin A consumption, and that this would have a beneficial effect even for the poorest households.

Potential to reduce VAD. Although the data are far from perfect, evidence suggests that in some states in the north with high VAD prevalence, mustard oil is consumed at all levels of society, even at low income levels, and thus biofortified mustard oil would reach those most likely to be afflicted with VAD. We conclude that biofortified mustard certainly deserves consideration as a pathway to reduce VAD in India, with the caution that several challenges to implementing the technology must be overcome. In the next chapter, we examine more closely whether investing in the technology to make biofortified mustard more available will be justified by the benefits to health and well-being among vitamin A-deficient populations.

Technology adoption. Indian farmers have been willing to adopt new technologies when promotional efforts and economic incentives make clear the benefits of doing so. Direct subsidies to producers, using a vertical integration model that extends from the farm to the processing facility to the distribution point, is an option, but subsidizing seed production through a market-based approach is less resource intensive and may have comparable results. It is also important to provide information to consumers so they understand the health and economic benefits they would stand to realize from consuming biofortified mustard oil. The information must be credible, and a reliable way to identify the enhanced product will be needed.

Notes

[1]The cruciferous plant family, to which mustard belongs, has long been known to have beneficial effects on health, including anticancer properties (Hecht 2000).

[2]Mustard seed is also used both crushed and whole as a spice, and as a paste in curries and fish dishes. In addition, the leaves of the plant are both eaten by humans and used as fodder (Nath and Lal 1995).

[3]Major oilseeds include copra, cottonseed, palm kernel, peanut, mustard-rapeseed, soybeans, and sunflower seeds.

[4]Shewmaker, Sheehy et al. (1999) found beta-carotene concentrations during genetic manipulation of *Brassica napus* (canola) of 314 to 949 µg per gram of seed (fresh weight), which, based on palm oil studies by May (1994), should lead to similar or greater concentrations of beta-carotene per gram of oil.

[5]Discussed in Bishai and Nalubola (2002).

[6]By some estimates, for example, there are more than 9,000 salt producers in India, many of them small scale.

[7]The diverse literature on how farmers learn about and adopt agricultural technologies is summarized in Feder, Just et al. (1985).

CHAPTER 4

Cost-Effectiveness Analysis for Treating Vitamin A Deficiency in India

Previous chapters have synthesized information on the extent of vitamin A deficiency in India and its consequences; strategies to increase intake, especially among children and pregnant and lactating women; and production and consumption patterns of mustard, which preliminary research shows can be biofortified with substantial amounts of beta-carotene. Chapter 1 presented data showing that in India, about 57 percent of children and 5 percent of pregnant women, mostly among lower-income groups, suffer from VAD. Although some progress has been made through supplementation, fortification, and food-based approaches, as described in Chapter 2, these efforts have not substantially reduced VAD cases in India, for various reasons. As summarized in Chapter 3, although biofortification of the mustard crop cannot be considered a panacea, it could play a role in some northern states that have significant levels of VAD and high mustard production or consumption.

In this chapter, we use a cost-effectiveness framework to evaluate the relative efficiency of biofortified mustard as a method of improving the vitamin A status of at-risk groups. We compare the costs and benefits of three population-based strategies: high-dose vitamin A supplementation for preschoolers (ages 1 to 4), fortification of mustard oil during processing, and biofortification of mustard oil with genetically modified mustard seed.

Because the primary goal of this project is to compare biofortification with alternative strategies for vitamin A dissemination, our analysis focused on states that either grow or consume mustard oil in significant quantities and have been shown to have a high prevalence of VAD (Table 4-1).

Table 4-1. States Included in Cost-Effectiveness Analysis

Mustard-Growing and Consuming States

Assam*	Madhya Pradesh*
Bihar*	Orissa
Gujarat	Punjab
Haryana	Rajasthan*
Himachal Pradesh	Uttar Pradesh*
Jammu and Kashmir	West Bengal*
Jharkhand*	

Mustard-Consuming (Nongrowing) States
Manipur
Nagaland
Tripura*

* Bitot's spots prevalence rates indicate VAD is a public health problem.
Identification of mustard-growing states is based on information in TERI (2006). Identification of mustard oil-consuming states is based on information in the National Sample Survey (2001), which identifies only states in which at least 10 percent of households consume mustard oil.

Our analysis focused mainly on the rural areas of these states, where the vast majority of the population lives, even though VAD is also prevalent among the urban poor (Kapil, Saxena et al. 1996; Gupta, Aggarwal et al. 1998; Kapil, Pathak et al. 1999; Khandait, Vasudeo et al. 1999; Ghosh and Shah 2004). Information on prevalence rates for urban areas is less comprehensive than for rural areas, where surveyors such as the National Nutrition Monitoring Bureau focus their efforts. Hence, we selected a subset of states with urban prevalence estimates (Uttar Pradesh, Bihar, West Bengal, Madhya Pradesh, Jharkhand, Jammu and Kashmir[1]), as well as the urban populations in two well-studied metropolitan areas, Chandigarh and Delhi, for urban-specific analyses.

The rest of this chapter details our analytical methodology, our principal findings, and the implications for decisionmakers.

Methodology

Analytical Framework

The analysis examines the three alternative strategies to alleviate VAD by calculating avertable disease burden in terms of DALYs and by comparing cost-effectiveness ratios in terms of unit cost per DALY averted.[2]

The DALY metric allows comparisons of alternative health strategies using a single index that combines information about mortality and morbidity. Following a similar analysis by Zimmermann and Qaim (2004), the total number of DALYs lost in a population through VAD is defined as follows:

$$DALYs = YLL + YLD_{temp} + YLD_{perm} \tag{1}$$

where YLL is the number of discounted life years lost due to mortality, and YLD_{temp} and YLD_{perm} are years of life with temporary and permanent disability, respectively, due to morbidity. To account for varying disease levels among the different target groups affected by the three strategies, YLL, YLD_{temp}, and YLD_{perm} are defined as follows:

$$YLL = \sum_j T_j M_j (1 - e^{-rL_j})(1/r) \tag{2}$$

$$YLD_{temp} = \sum_k \sum_j T_j I_{kj} D_{kj} (1 - e^{-rd_{kj}})(1/r) \tag{3}$$

$$YLD_{perm} = \sum_l \sum_j T_j I_{lj} D_{lj} (1 - e^{-rL_j})(1/r) \tag{4}$$

where T_j is the total number of people in the target group j, M_j is the mortality rate associated with VAD, and L_j is the average remaining life expectancy. I_{kj} is the incidence rate of temporary sequela k, D_{kj} is the corresponding disability weight, and d_{kj} is the duration of the disability. I_{lj} is the incidence rate of permanent sequela l, and r is the discount rate for future life years. This analysis does not include age weighting.

The impact of a specific intervention to reduce VAD is calculated as the DALYs averted due to the intervention. The total number of DALYs averted is defined as follows:

$$DALYs_{averted} = YLL_{averted} + YLD_{temp,averted} + YLD_{perm,averted} \qquad (5)$$

such that:

$$YLL_{averted} = \sum_j T_j M_j^{averted} (1 - e^{-rL_j})(1/r) \qquad (6)$$

$$YLD_{temp,averted} = \sum_k \sum_j T_j I_{kj}^{averted} D_{kj} (1 - e^{-rt})(1/r) \qquad (7)$$

$$YLD_{perm,averted} = \sum_l \sum_j T_j I_{lj}^{averted} D_{lj} (1 - e^{-rL_j})(1/r) \qquad (8)$$

where $M_j^{averted}$ is the reduction in the mortality rate of the target group due to the intervention, and $I_{kj}^{averted}$ and $I_{lj}^{averted}$ are reductions in the morbidity rates of temporary and permanent sequelae, respectively. The parameter t is the duration of the intervention.

This framework contains several important assumptions. We assumed that the reduction of temporary sequelae within the target group lasted only as long as the duration of the intervention. In the context of VAD, this assumption is based on the rationale that an individual with clinical deficiency would continue to suffer from morbidity such as Bitot's spots or night blindness unless the intervention were in place. However, permanent sequelae, such as childhood blindness, are averted for the lifetime of the treated individual. In addition, we also assumed that individuals who would have died if not for the intervention would live for their remaining life expectancy. Lastly, we assumed that an intervention lasting less than two years for a cohort of children aged 0-4 would not reduce the mortality rate nor permanent sequelae.

We evaluated the efficacy of a particular intervention according to the ratio of its total cost to its total effectiveness over a 20-year time frame. Effectiveness is expressed in terms of averted cases of sequelae, averted deaths, or averted DALYs. A greater cost-effectiveness ratio indicates a higher cost per unit of health gained. Hence, a high ratio indicates low efficiency or lesser cost-effectiveness, and a low ratio indicates the opposite. We also attribute a monetary value to a DALY to calculate internal rates of return. The monetary value chosen is annual per capita income in current Rs. for the year 2003–2004 (Chandigarh National Informatics Centre 2007). The goal of this approach is to estimate a convenient metric for economic analysis, not to quantify the intrinsic value of life. Therefore, the internal rate of return estimates should be interpreted carefully. They are not predicted rates of return of investment, but rather an index that is scaled with the average local living standard by which to judge the comparative efficacy of an intervention.

Biofortified mustard is still in the R&D stage and has not undergone field trials for either production or consumption. Hence, in this ex ante framework, parameters such as program costs and reductions in mortality and morbidity rates are not yet known and must be estimated based on assumptions about health services, agricultural and food production, and delivery systems in India. We modeled our analyses based on interviews with experts in VAD and mustard production and consumption in India, and also drew from recent demographic data.

Data

Our analysis used state-level data to estimate state-specific mustard oil consumption among young children and women of reproductive age, as well as rates of effectiveness in reducing morbidity and mortality associated with VAD. The list of data and sources appears in Table 4-2.

We calculated all results in units of both Rs. and US$, using the exchange rate of Rs. 40 = US$1.

Table 4-2. Data Sources for Cost-Effectiveness Analysis

Data	Source
Population size	India Census 2001
Health worker absenteeism	Chaudhury, Hammer et al. 2006
Baseline average daily vitamin A intake among children	Toteja and Singh 2004
Baseline average daily vitamin A intake among pregnant and lactating women	NNMB 2002
Mean daily intake of fats and oils	NNMB 1999

Monthly consumption of mustard oil per person per rural household	National Sample Survey 2001
Bitot's spots prevalence (rural)	Chakravarty and Ghosh 2000; National Institute of Nutrition 2001; Toteja, Singh et al. 2001; National Nutrition Monitoring Bureau 2002, 2003b
Bitot's spots prevalence (select urban)	Fakhir, Srivastava et al. 1993; Kapil, Saxena et al. 1996; Toteja, Singh et al. 2001; Swami, Thakur et al. 2002; Toteja and Singh 2004; Feldon, Bahl et al. 2005
Childhood night blindness prevalence (rural)	Toteja, Singh et al. 2001; TERI 2006
Childhood night blindness prevalence (select urban)	Kapil, Saxena et al. 1996; Gupta, Aggarwal et al. 1998; The Energy and Resource Institute 2006
Maternal night blindness prevalence (rural)	International Institute for Population Sciences 2000
Maternal night blindness prevalence (select urban)	International Institute for Population Sciences 2000
Fertility rate	Office of Registrar General India 2003
Crude birth rate	Office of Registrar General India 2003
Maternal mortality ratio	National Commission on Macroeconomics and Health 2005
Crude death rate	Office of Registrar General India 2003
Life expectancy	Office of Registrar General India 2003

We analyzed three interventions: (1) high-dose vitamin A supplementation for preschoolers (1 to 4 years old); (2) fortification of mustard oil; and (3) biofortification of mustard oil with GM mustard seed.

High-Dose Vitamin A Supplementation

This analysis considered a massive-dose supplementation program providing semiannual doses of 2,00,000 IUs only to children ages 1 through 4. These years were chosen in part because preschool children are not only more responsive to high-potency vitamin A supplementation than older children, but also more susceptible to corneal xerophthalmia (West and Darnton-Hill 2001).[3] We excluded infants younger than 6 months because vitamin A supplementation, either directly or indirectly through maternal provision, has generally not been shown to benefit early infant survival (Daulaire, Starbuck et al. 1992; West Jr., Katz et al. 1995; WHO/ CHD Immunization-Linked Vitamin A Supplementation Study Group 1998; Katz, West et al. 2000).

We considered a vitamin A supplementation program lasting 20 years. Averted DALYs were calculated based on avoided disability due to clinically apparent VAD morbidity, and avoided mortality due to subclinical and clinical VAD.

Averted morbidity includes cases of Bitot's spots and night blindness during the intervention, as well as lifetime disability due to blindness.[4] Bitot's spots and night blindness were treated as temporary diseases, the durations of which are taken at one year to avoid inflation of DALYs.[5, 6] For blindness, we conservatively assumed that the prevalence of corneal xerophthalmia cases is one-tenth the prevalence of Bitot's spots (see Rao, Klontz et al. 1961; Swaminathan, Susheela et al. 1970; Solon, Fernandez et al. 1979; Cohen, Rahman et al. 1987; Rahmathullah, Underwood et al. 1990; Swami, Thakur et al. 2002), and without treatment, one-half of all corneal cases lead to blindness (West Jr. and Darnton-Hill 2001). DALYs were calculated as the sum of disability due to Bitot's spots, night blindness, and blindness multiplied by their respective treatment effectiveness rates.

Because we lacked baseline information on the marginal effectiveness of vitamin A supplementation in India, we instead used a range of values reported in the literature. At the low end, we assumed a 26 percent reduction of Bitot's spots, 46 percent reduction in night blindness, and 43 percent reduction in blindness (Cohen, Rahman et al. 1987).[7] At the high end, we assumed a 75 percent effectiveness for preventing Bitot's spots and blindness, based on sufficient but incomplete coverage as well as some dosage inadequacy (West Jr. and Darnton-Hill 2001; West Jr. and Sommer 2002), and we assumed 100 percent elimination of night blindness (Sinha and Bang 1976).[8]

As discussed in Chapter 2, the level of mortality avoided because of supplementation is contentious. Thus, we assumed a range from 10 percent (World Bank 1993; Awasthi, Peto et al. 2007) to 23 percent (Beaton, Martorell et al. 1994). Avoided mortality was converted to DALYs by multiplying the number of deaths averted by life expectancy.

Costs were calculated by multiplying the number of 1- to 4-year-old children by per capita costs. Per capita costs were estimated at Rs. 1.98–2.58 (US$0.05–0.07) per child per year. These estimates included the cost of two doses of vitamin A per year, shipping, storage, delivery, and wastage (Anand, Sankar et al. 2004). We also included an additional cost of Rs. 3.33 (US$0.08) per child per year to account for training, promotional and educational materials, and program monitoring and evaluation (Micronutrient Initiative 2006), for a total of Rs. 5.31–5.91 (US$0.13–0.15).[9] India's supplementation program is implemented through the existing primary health care infrastructure (ICMR 2004). Because village-level health subcenters serve only a proportion of the population in each state, we stratified our analyses according to health subcenter coverage using statewide subcenter data published by the National Rural Health Mission (2006). We also adjusted these coverage estimates according to the rate of health worker absenteeism (Chaudhury, Hammer et al. 2006).[10] For populations without access to a public health subcenter, we estimated the supplementation cost at Rs. 23 (US$0.57) per child per year, which includes the cost of expanding subcenter coverage (Lakshman 2006). We did not consider costs for startup, program infrastructure, or other fixed costs, and the two strategies were not considered to have different effectiveness rates.

Fortification of Mustard Oil with Vitamin A

As in the analysis for supplementation, the cost-effectiveness of mustard oil fortification was calculated in terms of unit cost per DALY averted for a four-year intervention. However, because fortification of a commonly consumed food item such as mustard oil benefits all individuals in a population, the avertable morbidity and mortality were considered not just for preschool children, but also among new and expectant mothers—another group at high risk for VAD (West Jr. and Darnton-Hill 2001). Population estimates for new and expectant mothers for a given year were based on age-specific fertility rates and female population numbers from each state.

We calculated morbidity and mortality efficacy based on current vitamin A consumption, improved vitamin A intake with fortified mustard oil, and RDAs, following methods used by Zimmermann and Qaim (2004). The RDA values for preschool children and for new and expectant mothers were estimated to be 400 μg and 775 μg,[11] respectively (Toteja and Singh 2004). The improved intake was calculated by adding current vitamin A consumption to current mustard oil consumption times a retinol concentration of 18 μg/g[12] and a vitamin A retention rate of 80 percent.[13] Mustard oil consumption among preschool children was estimated based on average rural and urban consumption data (kg/month/person/household) (NNMB 1999; NSS 2001). Current vitamin A consumption for children (Toteja and Singh 2004)[14] and for new and expectant mothers (NNMB 2002)[15] was scaled down because it was assumed that the poorest segments of a population, those most likely to suffer from VAD, tend to consume less mustard oil per person than the average[16] (NSS 2001).

DALYs from averted morbidity and mortality for the preschool children were calculated as in the supplementation analysis. For new and expectant mothers, only disability from night blindness was considered,[17] and we assumed that the intervention prevented death among a different set of women each year. Additionally, we assumed that fortified mustard was available in the same proportion for all consumers. In other words, if a certain percentage of mustard oil in a state is fortified, then the mustard oil consumed by all consumers is fortified at the same percentage, regardless of the individual's vitamin A status.

The costs included the cost for the fortification process itself, as well as other costs to prevent vitamin A degradation and ensure product quality, such as bottling and quality control. We assumed that all mustard oil consumed was required to be fortified. Given the variation in the reported costs of fortification in India, we considered a range from Rs. 0.045 (US$0.001) (Micronutrient Initiative 2006) to Rs. 0.22 (US$0.005) per kg oil[18] (Nicholas Piramal India Limited 2006). We included an additional cost of Rs. 0.062 (US$0.002) per kg to account for training, promotional and educational materials, and program monitoring and evaluation (Micronutrient Initiative 2006). Because vitamin A fortificant degrades readily when exposed to light, the costs of bottling in opaque containers was also considered. We lacked information on the cost of opaque bottling, so the cost of bottling water was used as an approximation, reported as Rs. 2.5–3.75[19] (US$0.06–0.09) per liter (Bhushan 2006). Since these costs were scaled to the amount of mustard oil fortified, the total fortification and bottling costs for a particular state depended on its total mustard oil consumption.

Biofortification with Genetically Modified Mustard

Since biofortification and traditional fortification are similar delivery strategies for vitamin A, their cost-effectiveness analyses were alike except for parameter adjustments regarding costs and vitamin A content. Based on field trials, we assumed that biofortified mustard oil had a beta-carotene content of 185 μg/g[20] (TERI 2006), of which only 71 percent was retained after cooking[21], and only 75 percent of the mustard seed that was pressed into mustard oil was biofortified[22]. Based on these assumptions, we calculated an effective concentration of 49.3 μg of vitamin A per gram of oil at the consumption level.

Costs related to the distribution and sale of biofortified oil remained the same as for traditionally fortified oil, since both would require bottling in opaque containers and presumably require similar regulatory, monitoring, and enforcement frameworks. However, there were no costs related to adding artificial fortificant, since beta-carotene would occur naturally in biofortified mustard seeds and the cold-pressed oil produced from it. Instead, we incorporated a one-time fixed cost of approximately Rs. 22.7 crore (US$5.6 million) to account for the costs of R&D and licensing

(George 2006). We apportioned this amount among the states considered in this analysis according to their total rural population size, and then also applied the same rate to urban populations. We estimated that these fixed costs amount to approximately Rs. 0.40 (US$.01) per person.

To prevent the escape of engineered genetic material into natural ecosystems, the growing of GM mustard on a commercial scale could require additional bioconfinement practices by farmers, as well as additional regulatory and monitoring activities (National Research Council 2004). However, cost estimates for regulation of transgenic crops in India do not yet exist because the policies themselves are still being formed, and there is a great deal of regulatory ambiguity regarding transgenic crops. The most comparable example is Bt cotton, which in 2002 became the first transgenic crop approved for cultivation in India (Barwale, Gadwal et al. 2004). Farmers and others involved in cotton production do not yet incur additional costs for producing Bt cotton other than premium costs for transgenic seeds. Since biofortified mustard is not expected to be sold at an additional premium and because the regulatory framework is still unclear, we ignored any additional costs of growing biofortified compared with regular mustard.

Sensitivity Analysis

Because of the uncertainty surrounding our assumed parameters, we conducted a sensitivity analysis using Latin hypercube sampling (LHS) to evaluate the robustness of our results (McKay, Beckman et al. 1979). LHS, a type of stratified Monte Carlo sampling, efficiently analyzes large numbers of input parameters by treating each parameter as a separate random variable. A standard Monte Carlo simulation randomly selects each input parameter from within a probability distribution function. In LHS, each parameter distribution is stratified into equiprobable intervals and each interval is sampled exactly once, without replacement. An input vector is then generated, composed of the random samples of each of the input parameters for each simulation. The efficiency of LHS arises because each value of every parameter is used only once. The model may then be run N times to directly derive distribution functions for each of the outcome variables. Because of the probabilistic selection technique, the results can be interpreted within a statistical framework. Studies have shown that LHS is significantly more efficient than simple random and fractional stratified sampling designs (see Blower and Dowlatabadi 1994). LHS has been used to evaluate models within the field of epidemiology (Blower and Dowlatabadi 1994; Sanchez and Blower 1997; Blower, Porco et al. 1998; Schuette and Hethcote 1999; Blower, Gershengorn et al. 2000; Tanaka, Small et al. 2000; Blower, Koelle et al. 2001; Currie, Williams et al. 2003; Blower and Ma 2004; Blower and Chou 2004; Schwartz and Blower 2005). We used LHS to examine the sensitivity of the model to the ranges of each parameter, holding the level of mortality averted constant because the level of mortality aversion is contentious and significantly affects the results. Thus, we report a range and confidence intervals for both a low (10 percent) and high (23 percent) mortality reduction.

Results

Our analysis estimated the effectiveness in reducing morbidity and mortality associated with VAD through three methods: supplementation for 1- to 4-year-old children, fortification of mustard oil, and biofortification of mustard seed. Each intervention was evaluated using a low efficacy (10 percent) and a high efficacy (23 percent) of averted mortality, and results were obtained for the number of DALYs and deaths averted. We also calculated the cost-effectiveness and an internal rate of return of each intervention. The results of our analysis are presented in Tables 4-3, 4-4, and 4-5.

Table 4-3. DALYs Averted for Each Intervention Over a 20-Year Time Horizon

	DALYs Averted		Cost-Effectiveness (Rs./DALY)	
	Low Efficacy	High Efficacy	Low Efficacy	High Efficacy
Supplementation	1,74,46,000	2,76,47,000	1,500	930
	(1,70,93,000–1,77,99,000)	(2,72,91,000–2,80,03,000)	(1,420–1,580)	(880–980)
with subcenters	44,40,000	70,85,000	330	210
	(43,54,000–45,26,000)	(69,99,000–71,72,000)	(320–350)	(200–210)
no subcenters	1,30,05,000	2,05,62,000	1,900	1,180
	(1,27,38,000–1,32,73,000)	(2,02,92,000–2,08,32,000)	(1,790–2,000)	(1,120–1,240)
Fortification	1,28,44,000	1,86,27,000	10,060	6,880
	(1,25,10,000–1,31,79,000)	(1,82,08,000–1,90,47,000)	(9,830–10,300)	(6,740–7,020)
Biofortification	1,49,54,000	3,36,65,000	8,410	3,660
	(1,45,95,000–1,53,13,000)	(3,32,01,000–3,41,28,000)	(8,140–8,680)	(3,570–3,750)

(95 percent confidence intervals)

Table 4-4. Deaths Averted for Each Intervention Over a 20-Year Time Horizon

	Deaths Averted		Cost-Effectiveness (Rs./Death Averted)	
	Low Efficacy	High Efficacy	Low Efficacy	High Efficacy
Supplementation	2,63,000	6,08,000	97,900	42,000
	(2,60,000–2,67,000)	(6,04,000–6,11,000)	(93,000–102,800)	(40,000–44,000)
with subcenters	68,000	1,58,000	21,400	9,200
	(67,000–69,000)	(1,57,000–1,58,000)	(20,600–22,300)	(8,900–9,500)
no subcenters	1,95,000	4,50,000	1,24,600	53,400
	(1,92,000–1,98,000)	(4,47,000–4,53,000)	(1,18,100–1,31,200)	(50,800–56,100)
Fortification	1,55,000	3,56,000	8,27,700	3,57,400
	(1,51,000–1,58,000)	(3,49,000–3,62,000)	(8,11,300–8,44,000)	(3,51,400–3,63,500)
Biofortification	2,83,000	6,53,000	4,35,200	1,87,800
	(2,79,000–2,87,000)	(6,47,000–6,60,000)	(4,24,800–4,45,700)	(1,83,600–1,92,000)

(95 percent confidence intervals)

Table 4-5. Internal Rates of Return for Each Intervention

	Low Efficacy (Percentage)	High Efficacy (Percentage)
Supplementation	82 (79–84)	104 (102–107)
with subcenters	163 (160–165)	195 (192–198)
no subcenters	72 (69–74)	93 (90–95)
Fortification	11 (10–11)	22 (21–22)
Biofortification	16 (15–17)	43 (42–44)

(95 percent confidence intervals)

Source: Author calculations

Discussion

As shown in Table 4-3, Vitamin A supplementation for the entire population evaluated, at Rs. 930 (95 percent CI: 880–980) to Rs. 1,500 (95 percent CI: 1,420–1,580) per DALY averted, is far more cost-effective than either fortification (Rs. 6,880 [95 percent CI: 6,740–7,020] to Rs. 10,060 [95 percent CI: 9,830–10,300] per DALY averted) or biofortification (Rs. 3,660 [95 percent CI: 3,570–3,750] to Rs. 8,410 [95 percent CI: 8,140–8,680] per DALY averted). Supplementation is more cost-effective in areas with existing health subcenters than in areas without and would therefore be quite efficient in reducing disease burden without requiring investment in additional health infrastructure; however, large sections of the population would remain at risk for VAD.

Biofortification is more cost-effective than fortification (Table 4-3) but only if there are no additional management costs related to biosafety and biocontainment of genetically engineered material. Because biofortification is assumed to have a higher efficacy than fortification (because of the greater vitamin A content of biofortified oil), we currently do not know which would be more cost-effective should additional management costs be included.

The cost-effectiveness ratios translate to internal rates of return of 82–104 percent for supplementation, far exceeding the internal rate of return of fortification (11–22 percent) and biofortification (16–43 percent). However, fortification and biofortification reach both mothers and children and thus have the potential to avert substantially greater disease burden than supplementation targeted at children only. Hence, of the three interventions, biofortification has the potential to avert the greatest amount of burden (Table 4-5). We estimate that biofortification could avert 1.5–3.4 crore DALYs and 2.8–6.5 lakh deaths, versus 1.3–1.9 crore DALYs and 1.6–3.6 lakh deaths for traditional fortification. In contrast, while vitamin A supplementation targeted at preschool children in mustard-consuming states could avert 1.7–2.8 crore DALYs and approximately 2.6–6 lakh childhood deaths, without expansion of subcenter coverage, these numbers fall to only 44–71 lakh DALYs and 68,000–1,58,000 deaths averted.

Estimates for each intervention exhibited significant variation among states and between rural and urban areas (Table 4-6), but overall patterns remained the same as those described above. VAD interventions were least cost-effective across all interventions in West Bengal and Himachal Pradesh partly because these states have lower underlying mortality rates. Interventions also were less cost-effective in urban areas because of their lower baseline mortality rates.

Table 4-6. State-Specific Cost-Effectiveness Calculations (Rs./DALY Averted)

Rural Areas	Supplementation	Fortification	Biofortification
Uttar Pradesh	400–500	9,100–16,400	5,200–9,400
Bihar	600–1,000	8,400–14,000	4,200–7,100
Assam	400–600	9,100–18,000	4,400–8,700
West Bengal	1,200–2,200	20,300–33,900	11,300–19,200
Madhya Pradesh	400–800	5,800–10,200	2,100–3,700
Rajasthan	800–1,300	9,200–16,500	4,000–7,200
Jharkhand	400–600	12,000–27,700	5,800–13,300
Orissa	600–1,200	5,700–10,700	2,600–4,700
Haryana	1,100–2,200	17,300–37,800	6,700–14,500
Gujarat	1,000–2,400	12,600–21,700	3,800–6,600
Punjab	1,300–2,900	19,300–43,700	6,400–14,500
Jammu & Kashmir	800–1,800	14,000–23,900	10,300–17,700
Himachal Pradesh	1,800–3,900	29,800–61,000	16,500–33,400
Manipur	600–1,300	11,600–26,600	4,700–10,800
Nagaland	600–1,200	8,600–15,100	3,500–6,100
Tripura	500–800	13,500–29,400	10,000–21,900
Pooled	**500–800**	**7,100-10,500**	**3,600-8,500**

Urban Areas			
Delhi	3,800–7,000	25,200–47,000	12,500–23,400
Chandigarh	3,400–5,000	31,400–58,200	12,200–22,600
Uttar Pradesh	1,500–1,800	16,800–27,700	9,400–15,500
Bihar	1,400–1,800	15,900–27,800	8,500–15,000
West Bengal	5,200–7,400	67,300–115,900	45,400–78,600
Madhya Pradesh	1,400–1,700	18,000–31,900	6,700–11,900
Jharkhand	700–7,000	29,000–66,700	14,500–33,200
Jammu & Kashmir	4,200–9,400	32,800–54,000	24,100–39,800
Pooled	**1,700–2,200**	**16,500-23,000**	**8,700-17,000**

Range provided is for low and high scenarios for lives saved due to improved vitamin A status.

Comparison of Results

Our estimates for the cost-effectiveness of a vitamin A supplementation program targeting preschool children are in line with estimates previously reported in the literature, at least for areas with subcenter coverage (Levin, Pollitt et al. 1993; Houston 2003; Caulfield, Richard et al. 2006). However, our cost-effectiveness estimates for people without access to functioning health subcenters (Rs. 1,180 [95 percent CI: 1,120–1,240] to Rs. 1,900 [95 percent CI: 1,790–2,000] per DALY averted), a situation that applies to around 70 percent of the population, are higher than these previous estimates. Because the earlier studies rely on ex post analysis of empirical findings rather than the ex ante analysis of assumed parameters conducted here, the discrepancy between our results and these studies may be due to the numerous assumptions in our analysis intended to err on the conservative side of avertable disease burden, as well as uncertainties about the cost of supplementation.

It is difficult to compare our findings on fortification with the experience in other countries, since few formal cost-effectiveness studies of vitamin A fortification exist and none exists for oils. However, based on the few studies that do exist, fortifying oil in India may be less cost-effective than interventions in other countries that use different vitamin A delivery vectors. For instance, Caulfield, Richard et al. (2006) estimated the cost-effectiveness of sugar fortification at Rs. 1,328–1,409 (US$33–35) per DALY averted and Rs. 40,260 (US$1,000) per death averted in Guatemala. Earlier, Levin, Pollitt et al. (1993) calculated values of approximately Rs. 241 (US$6) per DALY averted and Rs. 9,098 (US$226) per death averted in current dollars. These differences may be at least partly related to the additional difficulty and cost of fortifying oil in India, with its large number of producers.

The only other biofortification analysis that could be compared with our findings was an ex ante analysis of golden rice to address VAD in the Philippines (Zimmerman and Qaim 2004). The results of that study suggested that biofortified rice had a cost-effectiveness ratio of Rs. 1,449–8,012 (US$36–199) per DALY averted, which is in line with our estimates. However, the authors estimated a much higher internal rate of return, 66 percent to 133 percent, because they assumed a per capita annual income of Rs. 41,467 (US$1,030) for the Philippines, whereas the values used in our analysis are much lower: Rs. 9,504 (US$344), on average.

In contrast to our results, other studies comparing vitamin A interventions have found that fortification can be more cost-effective than supplementation. Phillips, Sanghvi et al. (1996) found the cost per high-risk person achieving adequate vitamin A to be Rs. 40 (US$0.98) for sugar fortification and Rs. 68–75 (US$1.68–1.86) for capsule supplementation in Guatemala, confirming previous studies (Dary 1997). Fiedler, Dado et al. (2000) reported that vitamin A fortification of wheat flour in the Philippines was more efficient than supplementation. Both studies, however, acknowledged that supplementation was more appropriate in settings where the fortified food product was not consumed in sufficient amounts. Edeger, Aikins et al. (2005) also found that vitamin A fortification was more cost-effective than supplementation but noted that both strategies deserve consideration in developing countries. Furthermore, Dawe, Robertson et al. (2002) concluded that although golden rice is more cost-effective than supplementation in the Philippines, it would deliver modest amounts of vitamin A and would be insufficient as a stand-alone strategy. Hence, the comparative cost-effectiveness and favorability of supplementation and fortification depend on the consumption patterns of the fortified food delivery vehicle, and the two strategies can be complementary.

Implications for Feasibility in Addressing Vitamin A Deficiency

Supplementation

According to the results of our analysis, supplementation is by far the most cost-efficient strategy to address VAD in India. However, as discussed in Chapter 2, implementation of a universal supplementation program in India has been problematic. After 30 years of implementation, the National Prophylaxis Programme for Prevention of Blindness has achieved coverage of only about 30 percent (IIPS 2000), despite refocusing efforts toward children 9–36 months old and linking the program with routine immunization.[23] Controversy over whether supplementation should be bundled with immunization, whether it should be administered during single-day campaigns, who the target audience should be, and even its necessity in India have further complicated improvements in coverage.

Evaluation studies have indicated that vitamin A supplementation programs are poorly implemented and have inadequate coverage in most states, largely because of inadequate and irregular supplies, poor orientation of the administrators, absence of nutrition education, and poor supervision (Vijayaraghavan 2006). The difficulties surrounding vitamin A supplementation indicate that a targeted, state-specific approach is necessary. The results of our analysis suggest a framework by which states could be targeted for additional supplementation effort based on the cost-effectiveness ratio, internal rate of return, and current levels of supplementation coverage. Conversely, further expansion of supplementation programs should be approached with caution in states where the cost-effectiveness ratio is high, internal rate of return is low, and coverage rates are relatively high, particularly if VAD rates do not indicate a public health problem. Among the states considered in this study that have childhood Bitot's spots prevalence greater than 0.5 percent, all have low cost-effectiveness ratios and high internal rates of return, indicating that additional supplementation coverage would be highly efficient. Of these states, Uttar Pradesh, Bihar, Assam, Rajasthan, Madhya Pradesh, and Tripura have first-dose coverage rates that are less than the national average of 30 percent. Hence, these states deserve high priority for additional investment in supplementation programs.

Our results show that vitamin A supplementation is especially cost-effective in areas with access to health subcenters. Improvements in training, supply, and oversight at existing facilities could yield substantial gains in health. The World Bank (1994) recommends additional strategies to further improve the performance of supplementation programs, such as (1) inducing health subcenter visits by marketing the supplement as promoting health rather than preventing xerophthalmia, which is sufficiently rare that people believe they are not affected; (2) distributing supplementation records to beneficiaries and tracking supplementation status; and (3) scheduling regular weeks or months for supplements to facilitate management and marketing.

Finally, by assuming that VAD prevalence does not vary with subcenter coverage, this study ignores the likely possibility that VAD is substantially more prevalent in areas without access to primary health care facilities. Though investment in vitamin A supplementation is still quite cost-effective in such areas, fortification could provide a complementary way of reducing persistent vitamin A deficits. Moreover, supplementation in this context addresses only the vitamin A needs of children and not those of the wider population, particularly new and expectant mothers.

Fortification and Biofortification of Mustard Oil

Though it can be less cost-effective in absolute terms, fortification of food staples has certain advantages over supplementation. Fortification provides a continual source of vitamin A and is more likely to result in a sustained rise in serum retinol levels (Solon, Fernandez et al. 1979; Arroyave, Mejia et al. 1981) and, consequently, sustained protection from anemia and infectious disease. Additionally, our analysis shows that fortification of mustard oil may be able to avert a substantially greater disease burden over supplementation alone, mostly because the entire population benefits. Because additional beneficiaries primarily include pregnant and lactating women, one might argue that the difference in effectiveness could be addressed by expanding supplementation programs to them. However, as noted in Chapter 2, this strategy is not advisable because a sudden, large spike in maternal serum retinol levels caused by high-dose supplementation may increase the risk of birth defects (Rothman, Moore et al. 1995; Berti, FitzGerald et al. 2000).

However, like supplementation, food fortification in India is not without controversy, as reported in Chapter 2. Critics charge that fortification is more costly for small-scale producers than for larger producers, who benefit from economies of scale. They argue that laws that require fortification raise expenses for smaller producers and can drive them from the market. Moreover, the legality of fortified food products is not entirely clear, since the Prevention of Food Adulteration Act of 1955 makes additives to food products illegal, and the current law has no exception for fortification. The act does have a labeling clause, which requires clear labeling of additives, and fortification programs have been exploiting this loophole. Still, it has been considered a hindrance to fortification programs and will likely soon be replaced by a new Integrated Food Law that establishes a legal mandate for food fortification and inspection.

Unfortunately, in India, no food has yet been proven effective for enhancing the vitamin A status of vulnerable populations, although mustard oil could be a more promising delivery mechanism than other products. Dary and Mora (2002) estimate that fortification of oil is reasonable in countries where average daily consumption is greater than 5 g. Of the states examined in this analysis, only Madhya Pradesh and Punjab fail to exceed this threshold. Consumption also is relatively evenly distributed among income levels, with the most economically disadvantaged people in both urban and rural areas consuming substantial amounts of mustard oil. The cost of the fortificant is quite low, at approximately Rs. 0.09–0.22 (<US$0.01) per kg of oil fortified, and packaging is typically a negligible portion of the purchase price in India (Singh, pers. comm.).

Fortification of mustard oil, and oils in general, also has several advantages over using other staple foods, such as rice and wheat, as vehicles. The Vitamin A compounds needed for fortification of dry foods are less stable and at least four times more expensive than oil-soluble forms (Dary and Mora 2002). Consequently, dry foods tend to have less fortification and must be consumed in greater amounts to achieve a particular reduction in VAD. Oils also provide greater bioavailability of vitamin A.

Fortification of mustard oil entails some costs, however. Vitamin A is light-sensitive; hence, a fortification program would require opaque bottling. Enforcement programs would necessarily monitor both the fortification and the bottling procedure, increasing the costs to the state. Moreover, as reported in Chapter 3, the vast majority of oil processing in India occurs among traditional cottage-industry ghanis and small-scale rural producers (TERI 2006), rather than in centralized facilities (see Chapter 3). Although larger extractors produce a growing share of the domestic supply, the dispersed nature of mustard oil processing could substantially compound the cost of effective monitoring and enforcement. In addition, residents in more than half the country do not typically consume mustard oil. Given the potential cost of ensuring that enough mustard oil sold is fortified and bottled correctly to reduce VAD, the variance in mustard oil consumption among states suggests that investment in fortification, or at least its enforcement, is not advisable for every state in India. According to our cost-effectiveness and cost-benefit results, investment in traditional fortification and monitoring and enforcement is most advisable in Uttar Pradesh and Madhya Pradesh.

In contrast, biofortification, because of its substantially higher effectiveness and slightly lower production cost, would be an attractive alternative to fortification for many states. Investment in biofortification has a favorable internal rate of return and cost-effectiveness ratio in most of the states analyzed, suggesting that a program to support, monitor, and enforce biofortification could efficiently yield substantial improvements in health in states where mustard oil is produced and consumed and VAD constitutes a public health problem.

Despite its potential, mustard oil biofortified via genetic recombination technology comes with a unique set of hurdles that fortification would not face. GM mustard seed, which contains provitamin A in the form of beta-carotene rather than retinyl palmitate, would slightly darken the pressed oil. Mustard seed in India is mostly cold-pressed and unrefined and thus has a dark color even in its unmodified form. Nonetheless, the difference may affect consumption, especially in urban areas where preferences may be different. Moreover, Indian consumers have yet to demonstrate an acceptance of GM food products, since GM agriculture is still in its infancy in India. Introduction of GM foods to the public may require additional costs for education and awareness campaigns, depending on initial public acceptance.

Attitudes in India toward GM food and agriculture have been mixed thus far. In 2006, India's Genetic Engineering Approval Committee, the country's main biotech regulatory body, approved 19 Bt cotton hybrids for domestic cultivation, bringing the total to 63 GM cotton varieties. The committee has also approved the import of soy oil derived from GM "Round-Up Ready" soybeans, after previously curbing the import of food and feed made from GM seeds. The prime minister and president of India have urged the scientific community to develop new nutritional crop varieties using plant genome research. On the other hand, the Indian Health and

Family Welfare Ministry has proposed rules under the Prevention of Food Adulteration Act to require labeling of all GM food and feed ingredients, even though the health risks of eating commercialized GM foods have thus far proved negligible. In October 2006, the Supreme Court permitted Delhi University to conduct field trials of a GM variety of mustard seed for research purposes after prohibiting the Genetic Engineering Approval Committee from granting new approvals the previous month. However, permission was granted because substantial work on the trials had already begun.

Summary

Efficacy. Because of its increased beta-carotene content, biofortified oil can more fully meet the RDAs of women and children than traditionally fortified oil. Consumption patterns indicate that biofortified oil can improve the health of children in many states and contribute to that of pregnant and lactating women.

Efficiency. Vitamin A supplementation is the most efficient method of improving the vitamin A status of vulnerable populations in India, followed by biofortification via genetically recombinant mustard oil and then chemical fortification. However, fortification and biofortification can potentially yield a substantially greater reduction in VAD disease burden because it would be consumed by a larger segment of the population, including new and expectant mothers. Because of its greater vitamin A content, biofortified mustard oil could reduce more VAD morbidity and mortality than both supplementation and fortification, by several-fold.

Implications. Biofortification of mustard seed in states with high levels of VAD and mustard production and/or consumption is an attractive alternative to supplementation and traditional fortification. Despite its potential, it is unknown whether adequate amounts of the seed would be planted and consumers would be willing to use the processed oil.

Notes

[1] Urban prevalence rates for Bitot's spots are drawn from studies within a single urban district in each state. They are as follows: Aligarh (Uttar Pradesh), Patna (Bihar), Howrah (West Bengal), Gwalior (Madya Pradesh), Ranchi (Jharkhand), and Srinagar (Jammu and Kashmir). We used the same prevalence rates for childhood night blindness for both rural and urban populations because of a lack of information. Prevalence rates for maternal night blindness were drawn from the National Family Health Survey (NFHS-2) (IIPS 2000), which includes rural- and urban-specific rates.

[2] As noted in Chapter 1, DALYs are a measure of healthy life years—the sum of the present value of years of future lifetime lost through premature mortality, and the present value of years of future lifetime adjusted for the average severity of the mental or physical disability caused by a disease or injury (Rushby and Hanson 2001).

[3] The 1- to 4-year-old age group was chosen from a practical standpoint based on data availability: the national vitamin A supplementation program in India concentrates on children 9 to 36 months old (ICMR 2004).

[4] The disability weight is 0.25 for Bitot's spots, 0.15 for night blindness, and 0.5 for blindness (Zimmerman and Qaim 2004).

[5] Duration is taken as one year because we used prevalence rates rather than incidence rates (Brenzel 1993; Murray 1994; Murray and Lopez 1996).

[6] Other sequelae, such as corneal xerosis and keratomalacia, were not considered because there is little information on prevalence rates.

[7] In the study by Cohen, Rahman et al. (1987) the reduction was significant only for night blindness. We assume a 43 percent reduction in blindness based on the reduction of corneal xerosis (X2).

[8] The results by Sinha and Bang (1976) are from a study that administered 2,00,000 IUs of vitamin A every 4 months rather than semiannually, as is the case with the other studies cited. Nevertheless, we assume 100 percent elimination of night blindness because it is the earliest clinical manifestation of VAD and presumably the sequela most easily prevented with supplementation.

[9] Estimates by the Consultative Group on International Agricultural Research and International Food Policy Research Institute suggest that the costs of supplementation are significantly higher, about Rs. 80 (US$0.98) per child per year (Neidecker-Gonzales, Nestel et al., forthcoming). However, their estimates are not directly based on Indian data, and they estimated labor costs using average per capita income and not the wage rate of the health worker, as was done in Anand, Sankar et al. (2004). Since wage costs are the largest component of supplementation, the wage costs used by Neidecker-Gonzales, Nestel, et al. are significantly higher than the wage rate of health workers, and there was some ambiguity in how they arrived at their numbers, we used the lower estimates and varied these in the sensitivity analysis.

[10]Chaudhury, Hammer et al. (2006) do not specifically investigate the absentee rate among subcenter health workers. Among the types of health workers studied, they find that absence rates vary only with type of health worker (doctor/nondoctor), with doctors more likely to be absent. We use the absence rates they report for ward boys because ward boys are the closest match among the types of health workers investigated to subcenter health workers (NCMH 2005), even though ward boys can have vastly different responsibilities from subcenter health workers.

[11]The RDA for pregnant women is 600 μg, and the RDA for lactating women is 950 μg. Because we considered these two groups as a whole, we assume the midpoint, 775 μg, as the RDA.

[12]We assumed a vitamin A content of 60 IUs/g fortified oil, as recommended by Nicholas Piramal India Ltd. 1 IU = 0.3 μg retinol (Singh 2006).

[13]Retention rates of vitamin A supplement during storage are more than 95 percent after 3 months and more than 92 percent after 6 months (Nicholas Piramal India Ltd. 2006). Because the supply chain from producer to retailer is relatively quick, and because rural households typically utilize mustard oil immediately after purchase (Singh 2006), we assume no degradation of vitamin A due to storage. Approximately 90 percent of oil consumed is used for brief, low-heat frying (Singh 2002). According to Nicholas Piramal India Ltd., the vitamin A supplement has a retention rate of 78–90 percent after five minutes of frying at 180°C to 220°C. Hence, we chose a conservative retention rate of 80 percent.

[14]Where possible, baseline estimates of current vitamin A consumption were sex specific as well as state specific. For states without baseline information, the population-weighted average of the pooled current vitamin A consumption was used in statewide analyses.

[15]The NNMB (Shewmaker, Sheehy et al. 1999) lists current vitamin A consumption for both pregnant and lactating women. Because we considered these two groups as a whole, we took the midpoint between the two estimates. For states without baseline information on current vitamin A consumption, the population-weighted regional average was used in statewide analyses.

[16]According to our analysis of consumption data published by the National Sample Survey Organization (NSS 2001), the poorest 20 percent of rural populations consume 69 percent of the rural average, and the poorest 20 percent of urban populations consume 67 percent of the urban average. Presumably, the poorest are also most likely to suffer from VAD. Overestimating the amount of mustard oil consumed among those afflicted with VAD would result in an overestimated effectiveness rate. Hence, to maintain conservative estimates of effectiveness, we scaled down the statewide average consumption by 31 percent and 33 percent for rural and urban populations, respectively, and applied the resulting rates to the entire population considered.

[17]Night blindness is the only sequela for which prevalence information among new and expectant mothers is relatively comprehensive.

[18]This cost is reported in terms of unit cost per volume oil. Because our consumption data were in units of mass, we converted the units assuming a density of 0.985 g/mL for unrefined mustard oil (Transport Information Service 2006). Nicholas Piramal India Ltd. is a private company in India that produces and sells vitamin A fortificant. The commercial cost of fortification that the company reports is presumably based on the market price.

[19]Again, we converted volume to mass by assuming an oil density of 0.985 g/mL.

[20]This concentration of vitamin A in biofortified oil is a relatively conservative estimate. In the laboratory setting, pressed oil from GM mustard seed could contain, on average, as much as 600 µg per gram of oil (George 2006).

[21]This is based on the retention in crude palm oil when used as a shallow frying medium at 180°C (Manorama and Rukmini 1991). It differs from fortification because of the chemical differences between a fortificant and expressed beta-carotene.

[22]The variety of mustard being developed for expression of beta-carotene is 70–80 percent of the mustard grown in India. For this reason, we assumed that biofortified mustard is extensively grown and mixed with seeds from other mustard varieties at this rate when pressed into oil.

[23]First-dose supplementation, delivered alongside measles vaccination, is higher and more consistent than subsequent doses and has varied by state.

Conclusions and Recommendations

India has the highest rates of vitamin A deficiency in the world. Although VAD rates have been falling over past decades, more than 2 crore (20 million) Indian children suffer from some form of VAD, resulting in about 3,30,000 deaths each year. In this report, we consider three main approaches to addressing VAD in India—high-dose supplementation, fortification of food products at the time of manufacture, and a novel approach relying on biofortification using genetically modified varieties of an oilseed crop. We make the following five conclusions and recommendations about addressing VAD in India using biofortification technologies.

1. The public health significance of VAD is underrecognized in India. The most significant challenge to addressing VAD is the lack of recognition of the problem. Recent advances in crop genetic modification have made it possible to biofortify mustard oil with beta-carotene, which is converted to vitamin A in the body; but without greater efforts to publicize the magnitude and importance of VAD by premier Indian institutions like the Indian Council for Medical Research, the National Institute of Nutrition, the Indian Medical Association, and NGOs, it will be difficult to gather momentum around any strategy to address the problem.

2. Supplementation, traditional fortification, and food-based approaches have been relatively unsuccessful. Traditional methods of supplementation, fortification, and food-based approaches have failed to reach the severely affected, for operational, social, and political reasons. Where public health infrastructure is available, supplementation remains a feasible option. But the current program reaches only about one-third of the children who need it, and coverage is low in states with the highest rates of VAD. Despite efforts by the government and NGOs, only about 1 percent of food in India is fortified with vitamin A. Lack of enforcement, resistance by producers to incur additional costs not borne by their competitors, and the dispersed nature of production and processing facilities of many common foods have impeded more widespread fortification efforts. Food-based approaches, such as those using home gardening and dietary diversification efforts, have not had much impact because of the low levels of consumption of animal products (including the fats necessary for the body to absorb vitamin A from vegetables) by lower-income households.

3. Biofortification can be an effective and cost-effective way of reaching people with severe VAD. Biofortification of mustard oil offers the potential of being a new, cost-effective tool to reach vitamin A-deficient households in remote areas. Since biofortification does not depend on industry cooperation (unlike traditional fortification), does not require an operational infrastructure for delivery (unlike supplementation), and can provide extremely high levels of beta-carotene to consumers (unlike many food-based approaches), it can sidestep the big hurdles to other methods of addressing VAD. From a technological standpoint, mustard offers an excellent medium to deliver vitamin A, for several reasons. First, a large majority of the mustard varieties grown are considered capable of being biofortified, and thus it may be fairly easy to introduce large amounts of biofortified seed into the market with little disruption. Second, mustard oil, which is the commonly consumed form of mustard, allows for the absorption of beta-carotene, which is fat-soluble. Third, biofortification allows the seed itself to contain the vitamin A, so even home processing, which is thought to be extensive, would produce mustard oil high in vitamin A. Fourth, consumption of mustard oil seems to overlap in many areas where VAD is a public health concern. Preliminary research indicates that only small amounts of mustard oil are necessary to significantly raise consumption of vitamin A, and that this would have an effect on even the poorest households. Our data suggest that biofortified mustard oil would indeed reach those most likely to be afflicted with VAD.

Although vitamin A supplementation is more cost-effective, fortification and biofortification have greater reach and thus the potential to avert a substantially greater VAD disease burden. Our estimates suggest that biofortification could have the greatest efficacy of the three approaches—averting 52–70 lakh (5.2–7.0 million) DALYs—because of its high content of bioavailable vitamin A. Supplementation should still be emphasized, especially in states where VAD constitutes a public health problem, such as Uttar Pradesh, Bihar, Assam, Rajasthan, Madhya Pradesh, West Bengal, and Tripura, with special attention to states with low coverage rates. Though relatively cost-effective in these high-deficiency states, traditional fortification is most cost-beneficial in Uttar Pradesh and Madhya Pradesh. Where cost-effective, fortification or biofortification could be used to reach vulnerable populations, especially those that do not readily benefit from supplementation programs, such as mothers and populations without access to primary health care facilities.

4. Important operational challenges of implementing biofortification will have to be addressed. Biofortification requires that farmers adopt GM mustard varieties and that consumers be willing to pay for mustard oil that may look different to them. These challenges are not unique to biofortified mustard and confront other agricultural technologies, including those specific to biofortified golden rice. Vertically integrated approaches that combine mustard growing, oil extraction, and targeting to high-risk consumers are likely to be very resource intensive. A lower level of investment is needed for market-based approaches that only subsidize mustard seeds, but these approaches may not have much impact unless the biofortified mustard varieties are adopted widely.

Two other points are worth noting. First, given that traditional fortification has had limited success in part because of producers' reluctance to incur additional costs that their competitors do not have, it is important to ensure that seeds and other inputs do not cost farmers more, or that higher costs are not passed on to processors or, ultimately, consumers. Second, advocates must consider outreach efforts that include the scientific community, medical associations, professional and government bodies, agricultural researchers and extension workers, and the public to communicate the costs and benefits of biofortified mustard.

5. The optimal approach for addressing VAD in India likely includes a mix of strategies. Because each strategy has advantages and disadvantages, and because cultural and socioeconomic conditions vary across the country, a combination of approaches may offer the best chances of success. In mustard-consuming states at least, biofortification could substantially reduce VAD. States that do not consume mustard oil, however, must continue to rely on supplementation to improve their vitamin A status or else develop an appropriate alternative fortification vehicle. Efforts to further test the technological and economic feasibility of biofortified mustard, possibly leading to commercial production, must take these broader considerations into account.

References

ACC/SCN (Administrative Committee on Coordination/Sub-Committee on Nutrition) (2000). *Fourth Report on the World Nutrition Situation.* Geneva, UN ACC/SCN in collaboration with the International Food Policy Research Institute.
——— (2001). *What Works? A Review of the Efficacy and Effectiveness of Nutrition Interventions.* Geneva and Manila, ACC/SCN in collaboration with the Asian Development Bank.

Achaya, K. (Ed.) (1984). *Interfaces between Agriculture, Nutrition, and Food Science.* Shibuya-ku, United Nations University Press.

Agricultural Biotechnology Support Project (2003). Final Technical Report. East Lansing, Michigan, Michigan State University

Ahmed, F., A. Azim, et al. (2003). Vitamin A deficiency in poor, urban, lactating women in Bangladesh: factors influencing vitamin A status. *Public Health Nutrition* **6**(5): 447–52.

Anand, K., R. Sankar, et al. (2004). Cost of syrup versus capsule form of vitamin A supplementation. *Indian Pediatrics* **41**: 377–83.

Arroyave, G., L. A. Mejia, et al. (1981). The effect of vitamin A fortification of sugar on the serum vitamin A levels of preschool Guatemalan children: a longitudinal evaluation. *American Journal of Clinical Nutrition* **34**: 41–49.

Awasthi, S., R. Peto, et al. (2007). Six-monthly vitamin A from 1 to 6 years of age DEVTA: cluster-randomised trial in 1 million children in North India. Presented at International Life Sciences Institute Micronutrient Forum, Istanbul, April 16-18, 2007. Available at http://www.ctsu.ox.ac.uk/projects/devta/index_html.

Bagriansky, J. and P. Ranum (1998). Vitamin A Fortification of P.L. 480 Vegetable Oil. Washington, DC, SUSTAIN.

Barwale, R. B., V. R. Gadwal, et al. (2004). Prospects for Bt cotton technology in India. *The Journal of Agrobiotechnology Management & Economics* **7**(1&2): 23–26.

Beaton, G., R. Martorell, et al. (1994). Vitamin A supplementation and child morbidity and mortality in developing countries. *Food and Nutrition Bulletin* **15**(4): 282-289.

Behrman, J., H. Alderman, et al. (2004). Hunger and Malnutrition: Summary of Copenhagen Consensus Challenge Paper. Copenhagen, Denmark, Copenhagen Consensus Center.

Berti, P., S. FitzGerald, et al. (2000). Field Test of Fortification Rapid Assessment Tool. Ottawa, Canada, PATH Canada.

Bhandari, N., M. K. Bhan, et al. (1994). Impact of massive dose of vitamin A given to preschool children with acute diarrhoea on subsequent respiratory and diarrhoeal morbidity. *British Medical Journal* **309**(6966): 1404–407.

Bhushan, C. (2006). Bottled loot: the structure and economics of the Indian bottled water industry. *Frontline* **23**(7). Retrieved 15 November 2006, from http://www.hinduonnet.com/fline/fl2307/stories/20060421006702300.htm.

Bhutta, Z. A. (2000). Why has so little changed in maternal and child health in South Asia? *British Medical Journal* **321**(7264): 809–12.

Bishai, D. and R. Nalubola (2002). The history of food fortification in the United States: its relevance for current fortification efforts in developing countries. *Economic Development and Cultural Change* **51**(1): 37–53.

Blower, S. M. and T. Chou (2004). Modeling the emergence of the 'hot zones': tuberculosis and the amplification dynamics of drug resistance. *Nature Medicine* **10**(10): 1111–16.

Blower, S. M. and H. Dowlatabadi (1994). Sensitivity and uncertainty analysis of complex models of disease transmission: an HIV model, as an example. *International Statistical Review/Revue Internationale de Statistique* **62**(2): 229–43.

Blower, S. M., H. B. Gershengorn, et al. (2000). A tale of two futures: HIV and antiretroviral therapy in San Francisco. *Science* **287**(5453): 650–54.

Blower, S. M., K. Koelle, et al. (2001). Live attenuated HIV vaccines: predicting the tradeoff between efficacy and safety. *Proceedings of the National Academy of Sciences* **98**(6): 3618.

Blower, S. and L. Ma (2004). Calculating the contribution of herpes simplex virus type 2 epidemics to increasing HIV incidence: treatment implications. *Clinical Infectious Diseases* **39**(Supplement 5): S240–47.

Blower, S. M., T. C. Porco, et al. (1998). Predicting and preventing the emergence of antiviral drug resistance in HSV-2. *Nature Medicine* **4**(6): 673–78.

Boileau, T., A. Moore, et al. (1999). Carotenoids and vitamin A. Pp. 133–58 in *Antioxidant Status, Diet, Nutrition and Health*. A. Pappas (Ed.). Boca Raton, FL, CRC Press.

Brenzel, L. (1993). *Selecting an Essential Package of Health Services Using Cost-effectiveness Analysis: a Manual for Professionals in Developing Countries.*

Washington, DC, World Bank.

Caulfield, L. E., S. Richard, et al. (2004). Undernutrition as an underlying cause of malaria morbidity and mortality in children less than five years old. *American Journal of Tropical Medicine and Hygiene* **71**(2 suppl): 55–63.

——— (2006). Stunting, wasting, and micronutrient deficiency disorders. *Disease Control Priorities in Developing Countries, 2nd edition*. D. Jamison, G. Alleyne, J. Breman, et al. (Eds.). Washington, DC, U.S. National Institutes of Health.

Chakravarty, I. and K. Ghosh (2000). Micronutrient malnutrition—present status and future remedies. *Journal of the Indian Medical Association* **98**(9): 539–42.

Chandigarh National Informatics Centre (2007). Chandigarh in figures: economic indicators–2005. Chandigarh Administration. Retrieved 13 March 2007, from http://chandigarh.gov.in/knowchd_stat.htm.

Chaudhury, N., J. Hammer, et al. (2006). Is There a Doctor in the House? Medical Worker Absence in India. Washington, DC, World Bank, mimeo.

Ching, P., M. Birmingham, et al. (2000). Childhood mortality impact and costs of integrating vitamin A supplementation into immunization campaigns. *American Journal of Public Health* **90**(10): 1526–29.

Cohen, N., H. Rahman, et al. (1987). Impact of massive doses of vitamin A on nutritional blindness in Bangladesh. *American Journal of Clinical Nutrition* **45**(5): 970–76.

Currie, C. S., B. G. Williams, et al. (2003). Tuberculosis epidemics driven by HIV: is prevention better than cure? *AIDS* **17**(17): 2501–508.

Damodaran, H. (2002). Trade seeks duty sops on vitamin A-fortified sugar. *Hindu Business Line*. 11 January 2002.

Darnton-Hill, I. and R. Nalubola (2002). Fortification strategies to meet micronutrient needs: successes and failures. *Proceedings of the Nutrition Society* **61**: 231–41.

Dary, O. (1997). Sugar fortification with vitamin A: a Central American contribution to the developing world. *Food Fortification to End Micronutrient Malnutrition: State of the Art*. Satellite Conference of the XVIth International Congress of Nutrition, Symposium Report. Ottawa, Canada, Micronutrient Initiative.

Dary, O. and J. Mora (2002). Food fortification to reduce vitamin A deficiency: International Vitamin A Consultative Group recommendations. *Journal of Nutrition* **132**(Supplement 9): 2927–2933.

Daulaire, N., E. Starbuck, et al. (1992). Childhood mortality after a high dose of vitamin A in a high risk population. *British Medical Journal* **304**: 207–10.

Dawe, D., R. Robertson, et al. (2002). Golden rice: what role could it play in alleviation of vitamin A deficiency? *Food Policy* **27**(2002): 541–60.

de Pee, S., M. W. Bloem, et al. (2000). Evaluating food-based programmes for their reduction of vitamin A deficiency and its consequences. *Food and Nutrition Bulletin* **21**(2): 232–38.

Dijkhuizen, M. A., F. T. Wieringa, et al. (2004). Zinc plus μ-carotene supplementation of pregnant women is superior to μ-carotene supplementation alone in improving vitamin A status in both mothers and infants. *American Journal of Clinical Nutrition* **80**(5): 1299–307.

Dohlman, E., S. Persaud, et al. (2003). India's Edible Oil Sector: Imports Fill Rising Demand, Washington, DC, U.S. Department of Agriculture.

D'Souza, R. M. and R. D'Souza (2002). Vitamin A for the treatment of children with measles—a systematic review. *Journal of Tropical Pediatrics* **48**(6): 323–27.

Edeger, T., M. Aikins, et al. (2005). Cost effectiveness analysis of strategies for child health in developing countries. *British Medical Journal* **331**: 1177.

Egana, N. E. (2003). Vitamin A deficiency and golden rice—a literature review. *Journal of Nutritional & Environmental Medicine* **13**(3): 169–84.

Fakhir, S., A. Srivastava, et al. (1993). Prevalence of xerophthalmia in preschool children in an urban slum. *Indian Journal of Pediatrics* **30**: 668–70.

Favaro, R., J. Ferreira, et al. (1991). Studies on fortification of refined soybean oil with all-trans-retinyl palmitate in Brazil: stability during cooking and storage. *Journal of Food Composition Analysis* **4**(3): 237-244.

Fawzi, W. W., R. Mbise, et al. (2000). Vitamin A supplements and diarrheal and respiratory tract infections among children in Dar es Salaam, Tanzania. *Journal of Tropical Pediatrics* **137**(5): 660–67.

Feder, G., R. E. Just, et al. (1985). Adoption of agricultural innovations in developing countries: a survey. *Economic Development and Cultural Change* **33**(2): 255–98.

Feldon, K., S. Bahl, et al. (2005). Severe vitamin A deficiency in India during pulse polio immunization. *Indian Journal of Medical Research* **122**: 265–67.

Fiedler, J. (2000). The Nepal National Vitamin A Program: prototype to emulate or donor enclave? *Health Policy and Planning* **15**(2): 145–56.

Fiedler, J., D. Dado, et al. (2000). Cost analysis as a vitamin A program design and evaluation tool: a case study of the Philippines. *Social Science and Medicine* **51**(2000): 223–42.

Food and Agriculture Organization of the United Nations (FAO) (2001). *State of Food and Agriculture*. New York, NY, Economic and Social Department, FAO.

George, C. (2006). Personal communication. Received 2 December 2005, by R. Laxminarayan.

Ghosh, S. and D. Shah (2004). Nutritional problems in urban slum children. *Indian Pediatrics* **41**: 682–96.

Gopalan, C. (1999). Nutrition and developmental transition: lessons from Asian experience. *NFI Bulletin* **20**: 1–5.

Government of India (1993). National Nutrition Policy. Ministry of Human

Resource Development, Department of Women & Child Development, Government of India, New Delhi.

—— (2001). Census of India 2001. Office of the Registrar General, Government of India, New Delhi. Retrieved 6 November 2006, from http://www.censusindia. gov.in/.

—— (2004). Agricultural Statistics at a Glance: Economic Indicators, chart 4.18(b). Retrieved 16 November 2006, from http://agricoop.nic.in/statatglance2004/ EcoIndicator.pdf.

Gragnolati, M., M. Shekar, et al. (2005). India's Malnourished Children: a Call for Reform and Action. HNP Discussion Paper. Washington, DC, World Bank.

Grotto, I., M. Mimouni, et al. (2003). Vitamin A supplementation and childhood morbidity from diarrhea and respiratory infections: a meta-analysis. *The Journal of Pediatrics* **142**(3): 297–304.

Gupta, K. K. (2000). Moving the Food Fortification Agenda Ahead in India. Manila Forum 2000: Strategies to Fortify Essential Foods in Asia and the Pacific, Manila, Asian Development Bank, International Life Sciences Institute, Micronutrient Initiative.

Gupta, M. D., M. Lokshin, et al. (2005). Improving Child Nutrition Outcomes in India: Can the Integrated Child Development Services Program Be More Effective? World Bank Policy Research Working Paper 3647. Washington, DC, World Bank.

Gupta, S. S., A. Aggarwal, et al. (1998). Vitamin A deficiency—still a major problem among the underprivileged population. *Sight and Life Newsletter* **1998**(1): 23–25.

Hagenimana, V., M. Anyango Oyunga, et al. (1999). The Effects of Women Farmers' Adoption and Production of Orange-Fleshed Sweet Potatoes: Raising Vitamin A Intake in Kenya. OMNI Research Report Series 3. Washington, DC, International Center for Research on Women.

Hathcock, J., D. Hattan, et al. (1990). Evaluation of vitamin A toxicity. *American Journal of Clinical Nutrition* **52**(2): 183–202.

Hecht, S. (2000). Inhibition of carcinogenesis by isothiocyanates. *Drug Metabolism Reviews* **32**(3–4): 395–411.

Helen Keller International (1999). Vitamin A Status throughout the Lifecycle in Rural Bangladesh: National Vitamin A Survey 1997–98. Retrieved 20 July 2007, from http://www.hki.org/research/pdf_zip_docs/HKI_VAD_1997-98.pdf.

Herrera, M. G., P. Nestel, et al. (1992). Vitamin A supplementation and child survival. *Lancet* **340**(8814): 267–71.

Hickenbottom, S. J., J. R. Follett, et al. (2002). Variability in conversion of ß-carotene to vitamin A in men as measured by using a double-tracer study design. *American Journal of Clinical Nutrition* **75**(5): 900–907.

Hopper, G. R. (1999). Changing food production and quality of diet in India, 1947–98. *Population and Development Review* **25**(3): 443–77.

Horton, S. (1999). The economics of nutritional interventions. *Nutrition and Health in Developing Countries*. R. D. Semba and M. W. Bloem (Eds.). Totowa, NJ, Humana Press.

Houston, R. (2003). Why they work: an analysis of three successful public health interventions. Arlington, VA, MOST USAID Micronutrient Program.

Humphrey, J. H., K. P. West Jr., et al. (1993). A priming dose of oral vitamin A given to preschool children may extend protection conferred by a subsequent large dose of vitamin A. *Journal of Nutrition* **123**(8): 1363–69.

IMRB International (2006). Personal communication. Received 16 November 2006, by R. Laxminarayan.

Indian Academy of Pediatrics (IAP) (2002). IAP Policy on Linking Vitamin A to the Pulse Polio Program. Indian Academy of Pediatrics. Retrieved 20 July 2007, from http://iapindia.org/vitapolicy.cfm.

——— (2005). Eligibility of children for vitamin A supplementation program. *Indian Pediatrics* **42**: 1009–10.

Indian Council of Medical Research (ICMR) (1995). Nutrient Requirements and Recommended Dietary Allowances for Indians. National Institute of Nutrition, Hyderabad.

——— (2004). Recommendation of National Workshop on Micronutrients Held on 24–25th November, 2003 at Delhi and Organized by ICMR on Behalf of the Ministry of Health and Family Welfare. New Delhi, Government of India, Ministry of Health and Family Welfare, Department of Family Welfare, CH Section, No.Z.28020/50/2003-CH.

Institute of Medicine (IOM) (2000). *Dietary Reference Intakes for Vitamin A, Vitamin K, Arsenic, Boron, Chromium, Copper, Iodine, Iron, Manganese, Molybdenum, Nickel, Silicon, Vanadium, and Zinc*. Institute of Medicine, Washington, DC, National Academies Press.

International Institute for Population Sciences (IIPS) (2000). National Family Health Survey (NFHS-2), 1998–99: India. Mumbai, India.

International Vitamin A Consultative Group (IVACG) (2002). The Annecy Accords to Assess and Control Vitamin A Deficiency: Summary of Recommendations and Clarifications. Washington, DC. Retrieved 20 July 2007, from http://inacg.ilsi.org/publications/.

——— (2004). *Vitamin A and the Common Agenda for Micronutrients*. Report of the XXII International Vitamin A Consultative Meeting, Lima, Peru, 15–17 November 2004.

Jalal, F., M. Nesheim, et al. (1998). Serum retinol concentrations in children are affected by food sources of beta-carotene, fat intake, and anthelmintic drug treatment. *American Journal of Clinical Nutrition* **68**(3): 623–29.

Kapil, U. (2004). Update on vitamin A-related deaths in Assam, India. *American Journal of Clinical Nutrition* **80**(4): 1082–83.

Kapil, U., P. Pathak, et al. (1999). Micronutrient deficiency disorders amongst pregnant women in three urban slum communities of Delhi. *Indian Pediatrics* **36**(10): 983–89.

Kapil, U., N. Saxena, et al. (1996). Assessment of vitamin A deficiency indicators in urban slum communities of National Capital Territory of Delhi. *Asia Pacific Journal of Clinical Nutrition* **5**(3): 170–172.

Katz, J., K. P. West, et al. (2000). Maternal low-dose vitamin A or ß-carotene supplementation has no effect on fetal loss and early infant mortality: a randomized cluster trial in Nepal. *American Journal of Clinical Nutrition* **71**(6): 1570–76.

Khandait, D. W., N. D. Vasudeo, et al. (1999). Vitamin A intake and xerophthalmia among Indian children. *Public Health* **113**(2): 69–72.

Kochar, A. (2005). Can targeted food programs improve nutrition? An empirical analysis of India's Public Distribution System. *Economic Development and Cultural Change* **54**(1): 203–35.

Lakshman, A. (2006). Personal communication. Received 14 July 2006, by R. Laxminarayan.

Laxmaiah, A., K. V. R. Sarm, et al. (1999). Impact of Mid Day Meal Programme on educational and nutritional status of school children in Karnataka. *Indian Pediatrics* **36**(12): 1221–28.

Lee, J., M. Hamer, et al. (2000). Stability of retinyl palmitate during cooking and storage in rice fortified with Ultra Rice fortification technology. *Journal of Food Science* **65**(5): 915–19.

Levin, H. M., E. Pollitt, et al. (1993). Micronutrient deficiency disorders. Pp. 421–51 in *Disease Control Priorities in Developing Countries*. D. T. Jamison, W. H. Mosley, A. R. Measham and J. L. Bobadilla (Eds.). New York, Oxford University Press.

Manorama, R. and C. Rukmini (1991). Effect of processing on ß-carotene retention in crude palm oil and its products. *Food Chemistry* **42**(3): 253–64.

Marathe, M. (2001). Fortified sugar: a potential vehicle for vitamin A fortification in India. Manila Forum 2000: Strategies to Fortify Essential Foods in Asia and the Pacific, Asian Development Bank, International Life Sciences Institute, and Micronutrient Initiative.

Mason, J., A. Bailes, et al. (2005). Recent trends in malnutrition in developing regions: vitamin A deficiency, anemia, iodine deficiency, and child underweight. *Food and Nutrition Bulletin* **26**(1): 59–108.

May, C. Y. (1994). Palm oil carotenoids. *Food and Nutrition Bulletin* **15**(2): 130–37.

McKay, M. D., R. J. Beckman, et al. (1979). A comparison of three methods for selecting values of input variables in the analysis of output from a computer code. *Technometrics* **21**(2): 239–45.

Merchant, S. S. and S. A. Udipi (1997). Positive and negative deviance in growth of urban slum children in Bombay. *Public Health Nutrition* **115**: 492–505.

Micronutrient Initiative (2005). *Controlling Vitamin & Mineral Deficiencies in India: Meeting the Goal.* New Delhi, The Micronutrient Initiative.

――― (2006). *India Micronutrient National Investment Plan 2007–2011.* New Delhi, The Micronutrient Initiative.

Miller, M., J. Humphrey, et al. (2002). Why do children become vitamin A deficient? *Journal of Nutrition* **132**(Supplement 9): 2867–80.

Mora, J., O. Dary, et al. (2000). *Vitamin A Sugar Fortification in Central America: Experience and Lessons Learned.* Arlington, VA, MOST USAID Micronutrient Program.

MOST (2004a). *Cost Analysis of the National Vitamin A Supplementation Program in Ghana.* Arlington, VA, MOST USAID Micronutrient Program.

――― (2004b). *Cost Analysis of the National Vitamin A Supplementation Program in Zambia.* Arlington, VA, MOST USAID Micronutrient Program.

――― (2004c). *Cost Analysis of the National Vitamin A Supplementation Programs in Ghana, Nepal, and Zambia.* Arlington, VA, MOST USAID Micronutrient Program.

Multiple Indicator Cluster Survey (MICS) (2001). *India Summary Report.* Delhi, India, Department of Women and Child Development and United Nations Children's Fund.

Munshi, K. (2004). Social learning in a heterogeneous population: technology diffusion in the Indian Green Revolution. *Journal of Development Economics* **73**: 185–213.

Murray, C. J. L. (1994). Quantifying the burden of disease: the technical basis for disability-adjusted life years. *Bulletin of the World Health Organization* 72(3): 429–45.

Murray, C. J. L. and A. D. Lopez (Eds.) (1996). *The Global Burden of Disease,* Vols. I and II. Cambridge, MA, Harvard University Press.

Nath, V. and C. Lal (1995). *Oilseeds in India: an Overview.* New Delhi, Westvill Publishing House.

National Commission on Macroeconomics and Health (NCMH) (2005). Report of the National Commission on Macroeconomics and Health. New Delhi, Ministry of Health and Family Welfare, Government of India.

National Consultation (2001). National Consultation on Benefits and Safety of Administration of Vitamin A to Pre-school Children and Pregnant and Lactating Women. *Indian Pediatrics* **38**: 37–42.

National Institute of Nutrition (NIN) (2001). *Annual Report.* Hyderabad, National Institution of Nutrition.

National Nutrition Monitoring Bureau (NNMB) (1999). *Report of Second Repeat Survey—Rural.* Hyderabad.

――― (2000). *Special Report on Food & Nutrient Intakes of Individuals.* NNMB

Technical Report No. 20. Hyderabad.

———— (2002). *Diet and Nutritional Status of Rural Population*. Hyderabad.

———— (2003a). *Assessment of Prevalence of Micronutrient Deficiencies*. Hyderabad.

———— (2003b). *Prevalence of Micronutrient Deficiencies*. NNMB Technical Report No. 22. Hyderabad.

National Research Council (2004). *Biological Confinement of Genetically Engineered Organisms*. Washington, DC, National Academies Press.

National Rural Health Mission (NRHM) (2006). *Annual Report 2005–2006*. New Delhi, Ministry of Health and Family Welfare, Government of India.

National Sample Survey (NSS) (2001). NSS 55th Round. New Delhi, National Sample Survey Organisation Ministry of Statistics & Programme Implementation Government of India.

Neidecker-Gonzales, O., P. Nestel, et al. (Forthcoming). Estimating the global costs of vitamin A capsule supplementation. *Food and Nutrition Bulletin*.

Nicholas Piramal India Limited (2006). Human Nutrition & Health—Fortification. Retrieved 15 November 2006, from http://www.vfcdnicholas.com/hnh/fortification6.htm.

Office of Registrar General India (ORGI) (2003). Census of India. Retrieved 31 October 2006, from http://www.censusindia.net/.

Roche/OMNI (Opportunities for Micronutrient Interventions)/USAID (U.S. Agency for International Development) (1997). Fortification basics: the choice of a vehicle. Information brochure. Santiago, Chile, Roche. Retrieved 13 November 2006, from http://www.mostproject.org/pubs2.htm#USAID/Roche.

Oplinger, E. S., E. A. Oelke, et al. (1991). Mustard. *Alternative Field Crops Manual*. Madison, WI, University of Wisconsin.

Osmani, S. (1997). The Abraham Horowitz Lecture: Poverty and Nutrition in South Asia. Nutrition and Poverty—Nutrition Policy Discussion Paper No. 16. Papers from the ACC/SCN 24th Session Symposium. Kathmandu, ACC/SCN.

Pental, D., A. Pradhan, et al. (2001). Breeding of oilseed brassica species by a combination of conventional breeding and genetic engineering. *Rapeseed-Mustard: At the Doorstep of the New Millennium*, A. Bhatnagar, R. Shukla and H. Singh (Eds.). New Delhi, India, Mustard Research and Promotion Consortium.

Phillips, M., T. Sanghvi, et al. (1996). The costs and effectiveness of three vitamin A interventions in Guatemala. *Social Science and Medicine* **42**(12): 1661–68.

Rahmathullah, L., B. Underwood, et al. (1990). Reduced mortality among children in southern India receiving a small weekly dose of vitamin A. *New England Journal of Medicine* **323**: 929–35.

Ramachandran, R. (2001). A programme gone awry. *Frontline* **18**(25). 8–21.

Ramakrishnan, U. and R. Martorell (1998). The role of vitamin A in reducing child mortality and morbidity and improving growth. *Salud Pública de México*

40(2): 189–98.

Ramalingaswami, V., U. Jonsson, et al. (1997). Malnutrition: a South Asian enigma. Malnutrition in South Asia. A regional profile. ROSA Publication No. 5. S. Gillespie (Ed.). Katmandu, UNICEF Regional Office for South Asia: 11–22.

Rao, B. S. N. (2000). Potential use of red palm oil in combating vitamin A deficiency in India. *Food and Nutrition Bulletin* **21**(2): 202–11.

Rao, B. R., C. E. Klontz, et al. (1961). Nutrition and health status survey of schoolchildren. *Indian Journal of Pediatrics* **28**: 39–50.

Rao, S., C. S. Yajnik, et al. (2001). Intake of micronutrient-rich foods in rural Indian mothers is associated with the size of their babies at birth: Pune Maternal Nutrition Study. *Journal of Nutrition* **131**(4): 1217–24.

Reddy, V. (2002a). History of the International Vitamin A Consultative Group 1975–2000. *Journal of Nutrition* **132**(9): 2852S–56.

——— (2002b). Vitamin A programme in India—why the controversy? *Sight & Life Newsletter* (Special Issue 55).

Reuters (2006). Indian court allows GM mustard trial for research. 14 October 2006.

Ribaya-Mercado, J. D., M. Mazariegos, et al. (1999). Assessment of total body stores of vitamin A in Guatemalan elderly by the deuterated-retinol-dilution method. *American Journal of Clinical Nutrition* **69**(2): 278–84.

Ribaya-Mercado, J. D., F. S. Solon, et al. (2000). Bioconversion of plant carotenoids to vitamin A in Filipino school-aged children varies inversely with vitamin A status. *American Journal of Clinical Nutrition* **72**(2): 455–65.

Rice, A. L., K. P West Jr., et al. (2004). Vitamin A deficiency. Pp 211-56 in *Comparative Quantification of Health Risks: Global and Regional Burden of Disease Attributable to Selected Major Risk Factors*. A. D. L. M. Ezzati, A. Roders, and C. J. L. Murray (Eds.). Geneva, World Health Organization.

Rodriguez-Amaya, D. B. (1997). *Carotenoids and Food Preparation: the Retention of Provitamin A Carotenoids in Prepared, Processed and Stored Foods*. Arlington, VA, John Snow, Inc./OMNI Project.

Rothman, K. J., L. L. Moore, et al. (1995). Teratogenicity of high vitamin A intake. *New England Journal of Medicine* **333**(21): 1369–73.

Ruel, M. and C. Levin (2000). *Assessing the Potential for Food-based Strategies to Reduce Vitamin A and Iron Deficiencies: a Review of Recent Evidence*. Discussion Paper No. 92. Washington, DC, International Food Policy Research Institute.

Rushby, J. A. F. and K. Hanson (2001). Calculating and presenting disability adjusted life years (DALYs) in cost-effectiveness analysis. *Health Policy and Planning* **16**(3): 326–31.

Saha, S. S., B. K. Sinha, et al. (2004). Post Harvest Profile of Mustard-Rapeseed. Faridabad, Agmarket.

Sanchez, M. A. and S. M. Blower (1997). Uncertainty and sensitivity analysis of the basic reproductive rate. Tuberculosis as an example. *American Journal of Epidemiology* **145**(12): 1127–37.

Schuette, M. C. and H. W. Hethcote (1999). Modeling the effects of *Varicella* vaccination programs on the incidence of chickenpox and shingles. *Bulletin of Mathematical Biology* **61**(6): 1031–64.

Schwartz, E. J. and S. M. Blower (2005). Predicting the potential individual level and population level impact of HSV-2 vaccines. *Journal of Infectious Diseases* **191**(10): 1734–46.

Sempertegui, F., B. Estrella, et al. (1999). The beneficial effects of weekly low-dose vitamin A supplementation on acute lower respiratory infections and diarrhea in Ecuadorian children. *Pediatrics* **104**(1): e1.

Sengupta, K. and P. Das (2003). *Cultivated Annual Oilseed Crops of India*. Kolkata, India, Partha Sankar Basu.

Shekar, M., J. Habicht, et al. (1991). Is positive deviance in growth simply the converse of negative deviance? *Public Health Nutrition* **13**: 7–11.

Shewmaker, C. K., J. A. Sheehy, et al. (1999). Seed-specific overexpression of phytoene synthase: increase in carotenoids and other metabolic effects. *The Plant Journal* **20**(4): 401–12.

Shiva, V. (2001). The mustard oil conspiracy. *The Ecologist* **31**(5; Supp): 27–29.

Singh, H. (2006). Personal communication. New Delhi, India. Received 14 July 2006, by R. Laxminarayan.

Sinha, D. and F. Bang (1976). The effect of massive doses of vitamin A on the signs of vitamin A deficiency in preschool children. *American Journal of Clinical Nutrition* **29**: 110–115.

Sivan, Y. S. (2001). Impact of beta-carotene supplementation through red palm oil. *Journal of Tropical Pediatrics* **47**(2): 67–72.

Solon, F. S., T. L. Fernandez, et al. (1979). An evaluation of strategies to control vitamin A deficiency in the Philippines. *American Journal of Clinical Nutrition* **32**(7): 1445–53.

Sommer, A. (1997). Vitamin A prophylaxis. *Archives of Disease in Childhood* **77**: 191–94.

Sommer, A., E. Djunaedi, et al. (1986). Impact of vitamin A supplementation on childhood mortality: a randomised controlled community trial. *The Lancet* **327**(8491): 1169–73.

Sommer, A. and K. P. West, Jr. (1996). *Vitamin A Deficiency: Health, Survival, and Vision*. New York, Oxford University Press.

Sridhar, K. K. (1997). Tackling micronutrient malnutrition: two case studies in India. Food fortification to end micronutrient malnutrition: state of the art. Ottawa, The Micronutrient Initiative/International Development Research Centre.

Stein, A. J., H. P. S. Sachdev, et al. (2006). Potential impact and cost-effectiveness of golden rice. *Nature Biotechnology* **24**(10): 1200–201.

Subramanian, S. V., S. Nandy, et al. (2006). The mortality divide in India: the differential contributions of gender, caste, and standard of living across the life course. *American Journal of Public Health* **96**(5): 818–25.

Swami, H., J. Thakur, et al. (2002). Mass supplementation of vitamin A linked to National Immunization Day. *Indian Journal of Pediatrics* **69**: 675–78.

Swaminathan, M., T. Susheela, et al. (1970). Field prophylactic trial with a single annual oral massive dose of vitamin A. *American Journal of Clinical Nutrition* **23**: 119–22.

Takyi, E. E. K. (1999). Children's consumption of dark green, leafy vegetables with added fat enhances serum retinol. *Journal of Nutrition* **129**(8): 1549–54.

Talukder, A., L. Kiess, et al. (2000). Increasing the production and consumption of vitamin-A rich fruits and vegetables: lessons learned in taking the Bangladesh homestead gardening program to a national scale. *Food and Nutrition Bulletin* **21**(2): 165–72.

Tanaka, M. M., P. M. Small, et al. (2000). The dynamics of repeated elements: applications to the epidemiology of tuberculosis. *Proceedings of the National Academy of Sciences* **97**(7): 3532.

Tanumihardjo, S. A. (2004). Assessing vitamin A status: past, present and future. *Journal of Nutrition* **134**(1): 290S–93.

The Energy and Resource Institute (TERI) (2006). Vitamin A socioeconomic review. New Delhi.

Toteja, G. and P. Singh (2004). *Micronutrient Profile of Indian Population*. New Delhi, Indian Council of Medical Research.

Toteja, G., P. Singh, et al. (2001). Micronutrient deficiency disorders in 16 districts of India. Part 1 Report of an ICMR task force study-District Nutrition Program. New Delhi, Indian Council of Medical Research.

Transport Information Service (2006). Mustard Oil. The German Insurance Association. Retrieved 14 November 2006, from http://www.tis-gdv.de/tis_e/ware/oele/senf/senf.htm.

Underwood, B. A. (2000). Dietary approaches to the control of vitamin A deficiency: an introduction and overview. *Food and Nutrition Bulletin* **21**(2): 117–123.

——— (2004). Vitamin A deficiency disorders: international efforts to control a preventable 'pox'. *Journal of Nutrition* **134**(1): 231S–36S.

UNICEF (2004). Monitoring the situation of children and women: vitamin A deficiency. Retrieved 22 August 2006, from http://www.childinfo.org.

——— (2006). Micronutrients—iodine, iron and vitamin A. Retrieved 7 November 2006, from http://www.unicef.org/nutrition/index_iodine.html.

UNICEF/Micronutrient Initiative (2004). Vitamin & Mineral Deficiency: a

Global Progress Report. Retrieved 20 July 2007, from http://www.micronutrient.org/reports/reports/Full_e.pdf.

U.S. Department of Agriculture (USDA) (2006a). Oilseeds: world markets and trade, Circular Series, FOP 9-06. Washington, DC.

——— (2006b). Production, Supply and Distribution Online Database. Washington, DC. Retrieved 27 September 2006, from http://www.fas.usda.gov/psdonline/psdHome.aspx.

——— (2006c). The Role of Policy and Industry in India's Oilseed Markets. Economic Research Report Number 17, Washington, DC.

van Stuijvenberg, M. E., M. A. Dhansay, et al. (2001). The effect of a biscuit with red palm oil as a source of beta-carotene on the vitamin A status of primary school children: a comparison with beta-carotene from a synthetic source in a randomised controlled trial. *European Journal of Clinical Nutrition* **55**(8): 657–62.

Ventatesh Mannar, M. G. and R. Sankar (2004). Micronutrient fortification of foods—rationale, application and impact. *Indian Journal of Pediatrics* **71**(11): 997–1002.

Vijayaraghavan, K. (2002). Control of micronutrient deficiencies in India: obstacles and strategies. *Nutrition Reviews* **60**(5): S73–S76.

Vijayaraghavan, K. (2006). Micronutrient Policies and Programs in India: Vitamin A Deficiency. Situational Assessment to Guide USAID Investments. Hyderabad, National Institute of Nutrition.

Vijayaraghavan, K., N. Balakrishna, et al. (2000). Report on Food and Nutrient Intakes of Individuals. Hyderabad, National Nutrition Monitoring Bureau.

Vijayaraghavan, K., M. U. Nayak, et al. (1997). Home gardening for combating vitamin A deficiency in India *Food and Nutrition Bulletin* **18**(4): 337–43.

Vijayaraghavan, K., G. Radhaiah, et al. (1990). Effect of massive dose vitamin A on morbidity and mortality in Indian children. *Lancet* **336**(8727): 1342–45.

Villamor, E., R. Mbise, et al. (2002). Vitamin A supplements ameliorate the adverse effect of HIV-1, malaria, and diarrheal infections on child growth. *Pediatrics* **109**(1): e6.

West Jr., K. (2002). Extent of vitamin A deficiency among preschool children and women of reproductive age. *Journal of Nutrition* **132**(Supplement 9): 2857–66.

West Jr., K. and I. Darnton-Hill (2001). Vitamin A deficiency. Pp. 257–306 in *Nutrition and Health in Developing Countries*. R. D. Semba and M. W. Bloem (Eds.). Totowa, NJ, Humana Press.

West Jr., K., J. Katz, et al. (1995). Mortality of infants <6 mo of age supplemented with vitamin A: a randomized, double-masked trial in Nepal. *American Journal of Clinical Nutrition* **62**: 143–48.

West Jr., K. P. and A. Sommer (2002). Vitamin A programme in Assam probably caused hysteria. *British Medical Journal* **324**(7340): 791a.

WHO/CHD Immunization-Linked Vitamin A Supplementation Study Group (1998). Randomised trial to assess benefits and safety of vitamin A supplementation linked to immunisation in early infancy. *The Lancet* **352**(9136): 1257–63.

Wolf, G. (1996). A history of vitamin A and retinoids. *FASEB Journal* **10**: 1102–107.

World Bank (1993). *World Development Report: Investing in Health*. Washington, DC, International Bank for Reconstruction and Development.

———— (1994). *Enriching Lives: Overcoming Vitamin and Mineral Malnutrition in Developing Countries*. Washington, DC, International Bank for Reconstruction and Development.

———— (2005). *Repositioning Nutrition*. Washington, DC, International Bank for Reconstruction and Development.

World Food Programme. (2000). Indiamix: Development of a low cost fortified blended food. The United Nations. Retrieved 15 November 2006, from http://www.wfp.org.in/publications/indiamixnew.htm.

World Health Organization (WHO) (1995). The Global prevalence of vitamin A deficiency. MDIS Working Paper #2, Geneva.

———— (1996). Indicators for assessing vitamin A deficiency and their application in monitoring and evaluating intervention programmes. Geneva.

———— (2002). *The World Health Report 2002: Reducing Risks, Promoting Healthy Life*. Geneva.

———— (2003). *The World Health Report*. Geneva.

———— (2006). Micronutrient deficiencies—Vitamin A deficiency. Retrieved 10 November 2006, from http://www.who.int/nutrition/topics/vad/en/index.html.

Yadav, A. (2006). Personal communication. Received 14 July 2006, by R. Laxminarayan.

You, C. S., R. S. Parker, et al. (2002). Bioavailability and vitamin A value of carotenes from red palm oil assessed by an extrinsic isotope reference method. *Asia Pacific Journal of Clinical Nutrition* **11** (Suppl 7): S438–42.

Zagre, N. M., F. Delpeuch, et al. (2003). Red palm oil as a source of vitamin A for mothers and children: impact of a pilot project in Burkina Faso. *Public Health Nutrition* **6**(8): 733–42.

Zimmerman, R. and M. Qaim (2004). Potential health benefits of golden rice: a Philippine case study. *Food Policy* **29**(2004): 147–68.